THE FAT FALLACY

The Fat Fallacy

Applying the French Diet to the American Lifestyle

To Linda:

Bon Appétit!!

William Clower, Ph.D.

WM Clower

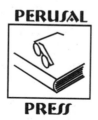

PERUSAL

PRESS

PITTSBURGH   2001

The Fat Fallacy is intended to be an enjoyable informational and educational supplement, not strict medical advice. The directions specified in this book should be balanced by consultations with your health professional.

Grateful acknowledgment is made to the following for permission to reprint previously published material: Oldways: Reproduction of the Mediterranean Food Pyramid, Latin Food Pyramid, and Vegetarian Food Pyramid developed by Oldways. Copyright 1994 by Oldways Preservation & Exchange Trust. Reprinted by permission.

CATALOGING-IN-PUBLICATION DATA
Clower, William
The Fat Fallacy: Applying the French Diet
to the American Lifestyle/
William Clower – 1st ed. p. cm.

Includes bibliographical references and index.
LCCN: 2001088313
ISBN 0-9709138-0-X
1. Nutrition. 2. Diet. 3. Food habits – France.
I. Title.
RA784.C56 2001 613.2
QBI01-200881

Manufactured in the United States of America
10 9 8 7 6 5 4 3

To *Dottie*

CONTENTS

ACKNOWLEDGMENTS

I cannot begin to list all the people whose kindness has been vital to the success of this project. The number of people I've met in stores, malls, and coffee shops is too large to include here, but all these incidental contacts have been important to the final product. With that in mind, I want to begin at home by thanking my wife Dottie for her help and support, and acknowledging my children Ben and Grace for tolerating my excessive attention to the computer screen.

I've been touched by the enthusiastic kindness of some dear friends in France: Peter and Jocelyn Dominey, Pierre and Regine Fournier, Remi Gervais and family, Claude Gomez and family, Michel Guyon and family, Pierre Jacob, Jean-Paul Joseph and family, Claude Lutz, Paula Usdin, Christine Usdin, and Francois Vital-Durand and family.

After returning to the U.S., many people graciously helped me with the ideas and implementation of this project: Bill and Retha Clower, Chris Cox, Beth Foley, Sandor Grossman, Clint and Diana Lathrop, Lisa McDaniel, Carrie and Tod McManis, Dorothy McMillin, Andy and Jen Nyland, Debra O'Conner, Kim and Alex Sobie, Shayna Smith, and Monika Wadman.

Introduction

We know the problem.

Only cigarettes kill more U.S. citizens than diet-related illnesses. Coronary heart disease, diabetes, and stroke top the unfortunately long list of weight-related problems, which represent 5 of the top 6 causes of death. Our incessant weight problems haunt us like a bothersome nag; carping in our ear about rolls and bulges, and the Barbie-like models that don't have them. In the other ear, experts clamor for us to latch onto their latest, greatest way to suck off, melt off, or drug off the fat. We respond to these insufferable voices by making resolutions, enlisting in health clubs, or taking on one more weight-loss regimen. But despite their panacea promises and commercial successes, the abundance of diet plans still has not inoculated us against our incredible obesity epidemic.

Quite the contrary. The number of overweight Americans only seems to expand by the year. Moreover, even academic nutritionists – the specialists in this area – deliver conflicting reports about where to begin. One news report warns that natural products like butter and eggs make you fat, clog your arteries, and then kill you. Two years later the opposite conclusion is stated just as confidently. Oily nuts, for example, used to be bad for us. Now they say walnut oil is loaded with a bounty of health benefits.

The problem: We're just too fat

It's not about ego or fashion. It's about whether we'll live another 10 years or another 50. The weight-related problems that dominate our health concerns include:

- Coronary artery disease, heart attacks, and congestive heart failure.
- Strokes and arthritis, particularly of the hips and knees: They've got to support that weight.
- Diabetes: The major cause of the "type 2" or "adult onset" variety is obesity.
- High blood pressure: Many people would be on far fewer blood pressure medications, or none at all, if they only lost weight.
- High cholesterol: To some extent, the genes we inherit from our parents influence our cholesterol levels. Nevertheless, dangerous cholesterol levels often return to normal once the body weight does.
- Sleep apnea.
- Breast, ovarian, prostate, colon and cervical cancer.

Riding on this scientific teeter-totter is the tiresome bicker of competing diet schemes. The most simplistic of these sings the praises of low fat diets – don't eat fat and you won't get fat. Another says, baloney, it's carbohydrates we should stay away from – eat all the fats and meats and cholesterol you want. Yet another accuses refined sugar of being the real culprit.

All these debates between the low fat, low carb, and low sugar gurus are well published, and each cites loads of statistics for his own side. But who do you believe when the only thing the experts agree on is that everyone else is wrong? What a mess. This confusion undercuts their credibility and creates cynicism among ordinary people who just want straight, practical advice.

I am not going to put an end to this debate. They will all keep pushing their point, like medieval scientists stamping about to prove whether the flat Earth rests on a camel's back or a turtle's. The ongoing diet controversy we see before us only points out that perfectly intelligent people can look at the very same data and come to completely opposite conclusions.

While they duke it out, what do we do? While the world waits at ringside to see if the low fat people are right and the low carb people are wrong – or vice versa – we need a solution that's right for us, right now. This is the point of *The Fat Fallacy*.

I lived in France for 2 years, ate as many sumptuous French foods as I wanted, and lost weight in the process. I was happily surprised. But I also felt duped when I realized that my American dietary dogma was dead wrong. The French break every rule our experts swear will make us fat. Wonderful creams, butters, and full fat cheeses (so much for the fat free theory) are spread daily onto fresh baguettes (so much for the carbohydrate free theory). And then there's the very essence of French foods, that blending of American dietary sins, the buttery croissant. Despite our brilliant science and dreadful predictions, their diet leaves them thinner and healthier than us, without even trying.

These simple observations are so overwhelming they leave us stunned. How can we try so hard and still fail so miserably, when they don't seem concerned at all and succeed anyway? They are clearly doing something right – something we don't understand. Given this, we have a few choices.

1. We can disregard the French and their diet altogether because they don't follow any of our dietetic strictures.
2. We can wait until we figure out why they don't get fat or heart-diseased and, once we understand it, make a plan.
3. We can simply imitate their dietary habits to get the same results they do.

The American dietary industry will advise you to blow off the data, it just can't be right. Someone from a research lab might tell you to wait until we understand why it works before you "try this at home." My own take is more intuitive, and shoots straight from the hip of common sense. If someone else has a successful dietary strategy, we can make it work for us just as well. *The Fat Fallacy* does a very simple thing. It applies the French diet to the

American lifestyle. By following these guidelines, you will drop weight on a long-term basis and learn to love your food again.

- Should you stay away from fats? No.
- Should you stay away from carbs? No.
- Should you agonize over the precise proportions of x to y in each meal, or calculate the number of hydrogens saturating the fatty acid chain? Again, no.

You don't have to have a Ph.D. in biochemistry or wag around a calculator to have a sound diet. You'll never see a French person feverishly adding up his meal on a calorie counter before enjoying a luscious chicken a la crème. With this dietary philosophy, you don't have to.

The Fat Fallacy diet works. It lets you eat *fats and carbohydrates*, increases the pleasure and balance of your diet, and decreases your weight in the process. Real simple. We've all grown up in the American culture of low fat, no fat diets. So the ideas in this book may seem to go against all the things you've been told. And they do. However, the evidence that the diet works can be found in the greatest trans-Atlantic clinical weight study in history. On our side of the ocean, 281 million Americans have been playing by the low fat rules all these years and getting fatter all the while. On the other side, 58 million French people nonchalantly spend their lives loving their food without our neurotic obsessions, without our obesity problems.

The Reader Replies: Monika

Well, I have good news. I read your chapters and was so immediately convinced that in whatever approximate way I could imagine I tried to implement the diet you describe. Well, I am down to 135 lbs from 146 last August, back to size 10 (from 12) and on my way to 8! And, boy, do I enjoy that cream on top of the whole milk yogurt!

Best wishes to you and your family,
Monika

Faux-Foods Quiz: What are faux-foods?

Food is wonderful. Paint thinner is not. You shouldn't eat that – or anything pulled off the shelf of a chemistry cabinet. The point is that a lot of the things we eat aren't actually foods, but accumulations of chemicals. I call them faux-foods (false foods), because their beautiful pictures and ads cheerlead us into thinking that they're really something you should eat. Faux-foods are more popular on American shelves than real foods.

Our bodies are set up to process things like beans, fish, fruits, chicken, nuts. If it gets partially hydrogenated gunk, or aluminum di-sodium lactoyl stuff, it just doesn't know what to do with it. This is a problem for your health, obviously, but it's also an issue for your weight.

At the end of each chapter, I'll have a quiz to see if you can guess these common products. And like any quiz, don't look at the answers in the back of the book. No peaking. Give it a good try. But because I'm basically a softy, I'll give hints along the way.

Ingredients

Water, sugar, partially hydrogenated soybean and cottonseed oil, sodium caseinate, natural and artificial flavors, di-potassium phosphate, sodium stearoyl lactylate (that's Ster – Oil – Lack – Til – Ate), polysorbate 60, carrageenan, beta -carotene coloring.

Hint

A very close friend of mine is an enthusiast of *The Fat Fallacy* diet, but has struggled to give up this faux-food. During graduate school, she and her family lived 60 minutes away from us. So when Dottie and I would go for a visit, we'd often stay the night. I loved those times first thing in the morning: the sun was still waking up, the kids were still groggy and cuddly, all the technology was off, and you could really relax in the momentary calm. This faux-food comes out during this peaceful time.

THE FRENCH AND THEIR DIET

1

The Big Fat Myth

It was a brilliant morning.
Even by 8:15, the early Key West sun had sunk its deep,
touchless massage through my skin and melted me into the
wicker weave of my high-backed chair. My wife Dottie and I
were enjoying our final breakfast of a conference on the neural
control of movement (a bunch of scientists, tanning and talking
about the brain and how it makes us move). Despite the delicious
April sun, the meeting was now over. Our suitcases were already
packed, so we only had to check out and head to the airport.

After chitchatting with colleagues over scrambled eggs
and coffee, we stood to go. A smallish French physiologist from
Lyon, also at our table, got up at the same time. Fate's funny like
that. Strolling with us as we left, he tossed his query out there
like a hopeful horseshoe heading for the stake. "You Americans
wouldn't consider doing your post-doctoral work in France,

would you?" Dottie and I stammered appropriate generalities, said good-bye, we'd keep in touch by email, and drove to the Miami Airport with our heads full of the thought. Living in France! This decision was a no-brainer. After many emails and two successful grant applications, we boarded a plane with two kids, two cats, my mother, and one-way tickets to work at the Institute of Cognitive Sciences for the next 2 years.

During our wonderful stay, it quickly became clear why Americans are so often confused by French attitudes, which sometimes seem to lurch straight out of left field. I realized, though, when my French friends acted like *I was the one* from another planet, that my American ways were just as bizarre to them. Being shocked by their strange views – and seeing their reaction to mine – became an exercise in self-reflection. There's no better example of this than diet.

The French *laissez faire* attitude toward fat and weight hit home on one of our first forays. We hopped aboard the bullet train and zipped across miles of elegant multicolored countryside on our way to visit friends near Lille, in northern France. On the first morning of our visit, our friend served the children (including my 4-year-old daughter, Grace) a shredded wheat breakfast cereal with a liberal dose of whole milk over it. "Whole milk!" I thought, "It's got all that fat in it. Don't they have 2% in this country?"

With such casual disregard for this major source of daily fat intake, you might think they'd be as large as cows. Of course they're not – our friends and their children (like over 90% of the French people) are small in size and not concerned at all about the non-issue of their weight. It never comes up because they're too busy enjoying their food. It gets better. On top of the whole milk in the cereal, they add a healthy dollop of pure cream. This happens every day.

It blares with a bullhorn that our cultural training has deceived us. We've had it beaten into our heads in drill sergeant fashion that we have to exercise! Watch the fats! Back off the carbs! Scrutinize the labels!   But even with all this dietary indoctrination, Americans are the ones with tar-baby obesity problems, who fret and worry about each pound, who drug themselves and starve themselves and have surgeons slice out their intestines to help them finally lose weight. At some point, though, we've got to ask ourselves why on Earth we continue to follow the same low fat/no fat dietary creed that brought us into this mess. Meanwhile, entire countries scratch their heads and wonder how our constant frenzy to control weight could produce such abject failure.

After returning to the U.S., I met our scruffy neighborhood lawn care guy, who asked me about the French license plates still on my car. I told him we had lived there and his eyes immediately glazed over. His thoughts percolated around in his brain, bubbling into a healthy reminiscent froth. Then he said, "I went to France … on a ski trip … for a month." He paused for another minute, clearly slashing his way, all sunglasses and ski poles, down the virgin alpine slopes. When he came back to us, out of the clear blue he offered, "There aren't any fat people there. If you find one, they're speaking English." I laughed. Unfortunately, it's all too true.

The purple puzzle piece

My mother came to stay with us for several months in France. She helped us manage our kids and home while Dottie and I were busy being overwhelmed with work, deciphering junk mail from the light bill, and figuring out the tortuous rules (and hand gestures) of driving among the French. Before she left the U.S., my mom was struggling to cope with the horror of buying size 14 clothes – doing the psychological shuffle. "It's okay. No, really. This is … you know … just where I am. People get larger when they get older. Right? Besides, I don't need to worry about cramming my fanny into those pants anymore anyway."

With all these rationalizations safely in hand, she resolved to relax about her weight while she was with us. "I'm just going to live my life and love it. And I don't care." You go, mom. Be defiant. So we all ate like the French, and had daily doses of high fat cheeses on our high carbohydrate baguettes. We indulged in creamy this and buttery that, turning a deaf ear to our guilty collective dietary unconscious. No worry, no self-denial, no counting up bits of food and saying, "Oh well, that's all I can have today."

Mom didn't even notice what happened. It was chilly during her stay, so she lived in baggy sweats much of the time. And she never saw it coming because she wasn't "dieting" or even thinking about losing weight. But by the time she returned home, my mom had gone from a size 12-begging-to-be-a-14 to a size 6, dancing around our living room floor with her arms up in the air like she had just won the lottery – in my wife's blue jeans!

If you believe, really believe, our standard American dogma of fat free weight control, this will sound like a dream – pure fiction. But it's not. We were shocked. She was shocked. My dad, well, let's say he was pleased with the new developments. She felt great without struggle, ate without guilt, and got thin eating sumptuous foods.

Now that I'm back home, I hear this same story over and over from people who have gone to France for any length of time. My neighbor across the street came over to pick up her daughter, who was having another sprawled out Barbie-fest on the living room floor with Grace – little plastic hamburgers, refrigerators, and Malibu sports cars everywhere. After my neighbor found out we had lived in France, she offered her own experiences.

"I went there throwing diet to the breeze," she said with a flamboyant wave of her arm and cock of her head. "I ate whatever I wanted and loved it! And you know what? When I came home I had lost 5 pounds!" I'd heard these stories before I left for France, but how can you believe them when the chatter of tabloids and "experts" all say how bad this kind of diet is for you?

It's a real dilemma. What do you do when you see one thing with your own eyes (the French diet just plain works), but hear another from your own experts (the French diet *just can't work*)? Our first response is typical. When observations don't come out like they "should," and we really can't explain what's going on, just ignore them. That's simple enough.

Blowing off the dietary habits of fat-ambivalent countries like France is a perfect example. That's why you seldom hear reports about how few overweight people there are in France, because the French eating habits are so different from ours. They eat all that fat, all those breads, with 3-hour meals late at night!

If our results don't agree with what we already know, there must be some other explanation. Notice that many dietician scientists, who cannot begin to explain why the French are thin and we are not, don't even ask what's wrong with our current dietary strategies. We cling to the faith of our dietary creed like an Alabama Baptist at a Darwin convention. It's right. It just is. We hold on, and don't question our beliefs because of one critical assumption: our fat free theories must, eventually, be able to explain away all those pesky thin French people.

But it's harder and harder to justify the tottering old dogma. The average French life span is longer than ours (2 years for men, and 3 years for women) despite our sterling medical system and despite the fact that they smoke like fiends (See www-nt.who.int/whosis to directly compare the health statistics of the U.S. and France). The most recent data from the World Health Organization shows that we are an incredible 3 times more likely to get ischemic heart diseases than the French.

Explanations, though, are hard to come by. Maybe it's the cheese they eat, maybe it's the wine they drink. Who knows? A close friend of mine, who is a biochemistry professor, actually offered that it's because the bread is really chewy and requires more calories to eat! We're clearly at a loss.

One scientific paper suggested that perhaps a high "folic acid intake" explained their good heath. Another shot-in-the-dark explanation claimed that their lack of heart disease might be due to "merely the consequence of having longer, warmer, and sunnier days and easier access to fresh fruit and vegetables." The author never mentioned the sky-high heart disease rates in sunny Florida, Texas, and California, where access to warm climate and fresh fruits is unsurpassed, even in France. Here again, our incredible tendency is to make up explanations so we won't have to abandon the ship that has brought us here. And the band on the *Titanic* played, all the way down.

Clearly, we're stuck in our stammering confusion – so much so that we don't even know where to point a blaming finger. It used to be that simple exercise was the scapegoat for our weight-related problems, but we can't fall back on that any more. A study in the *Journal of the American Medical Association* reported the activity and obesity rates from 1991 to 1998. During that time, the number of U.S. states with more than a 15% obesity rate jumped a whopping 825%, from 4 to 37.

What do you suppose happened to activity rates over this same interval? You might guess that we're getting fatter because we're less active, sitting around on the couch like Jabba the Hut with a remote. But even coming on the heels of the "fitness explosion" of the 70's and 80's, this study found that many people were more active than ever. In fact, the percentage of people who were "intense" about their workouts increased from 8.7 to 13.6! Intense exercise increased. Americans got steadily fatter anyway. The bottom line is that exercise is only one part of a complex solution – one that still eludes us.

So why are we so confused? We're not confused because of bad scientific research, but because we've been thinking about the problem all wrong. If you're working on a puzzle that's basically green, and you reach into the bag and pull out a purple piece, you'll look at it like we look at the French diet. You'll scratch your head. You might even suggest it doesn't belong in this puzzle at all. The confusion comes because you have no clue how it could possibly fit into the beautiful green picture you've created. With one purple puzzle piece in your hand and a great big green puzzle spread out on the board in front of you, you essentially have two choices. Either throw away this wonderful green elaboration you've invested so much time and energy on, or trash those pesky purple facts that just don't fit.

The American dietary establishment has no credible way to explain why the French diet doesn't produce a country full of heart-diseased fat people (like ours), but keeps droning the same fat free mantra, disregarding those disagreeable data. Maybe if they ignore it long enough, it'll go away. But then again, maybe not.

Good for your weight, but also your health

My mom has a close friend who is a nurse. When he found out she was eating so much milk fat in France, he almost had a heart attack. What about her cholesterol! We all know how bad that is for your arteries! His blood pressure soared in sympathy. But when she returned home and went to the doctor, her cholesterol count was fine. All that milk fat didn't disturb her doctor one bit – once he saw that it didn't put her at any risk. In fact, Dottie's mom also came for an extended visit in our den of dietary decadence. After she returned to the U.S. and went to her doctor, she found that her "good" cholesterol held steady and her "bad" cholesterol actually decreased.

How many examples do we need before we just believe our own eyes? The French diet doesn't make you fat or unhealthy. For my part, I never had my cholesterol tested before I left. But after almost 2 full years of enjoying wonderful foods, eating the rich butterfat from around the cream container with a spoon, and scoffing openly in front of God and everybody about how the low fat, taste-free food religion is wrong, I returned home and went to the doctor. My "good" cholesterol was high (56; it should be over 35), my "bad" cholesterol was low (110; it should be under 130). The only thing that blipped on my chart was the indicator for heart disease. This reading informed me about my *unusually low risk* of having a heart attack! The doctor just closed his eyes, shook his head, and chuckled. By the way, I never exercised a day in France.

This isn't to say that the French have no distinctions around the health effects of fats. All fats aren't created equal; some are definitely better for you than others. I first learned about this from chef Claude Lutz. Some 23 years ago, he had gone to apprentice under one of France's finest chefs. Then he came back home to run his own place. He'd obviously worked very hard and acquired a good reputation along the way.

We talked and gestured over our small black coffees for more than an hour: about food and the French, food and the Americans, body image, etc. "Sure," he said, "it's mostly the young girls who think about their weight in the spring and forget it in the fall. Interest waxes and wanes depending on whether they're in the same room with their bikinis." No one, though, doubts that creams and cheeses and butters are a staple health food. On the other hand, he wagged his finger at me, the fat of some animal meats will kill you. This was not the first nor the last time I'd heard this.

Obesity cascades into numerous diseases

According to the Calorie Control Council, increasing your weight increases a list of health problems.

Your % Overweight	Increased Risk of Disease
• 20% overweight	Death by any cause (20%)
	Heart disease (25%)
	Stroke (10%)
	Diabetes (50%)
	Gall bladder disease (40%)
• 40% overweight	Death by any cause (55%)
	Heart disease (70%)
	Stroke (75%)
	Diabetes (400%)
• For every 10% more	Heart disease (+20%)

See also:
www.american.edu/projects/mandala/TED/olestra.htm

The bad fats, well known to the French chefs and ordinary people, are not counted by the number of hydrogens saturating the fatty acid chain. This is way too beaker-complicated for an older country with a long cultural tradition. The bad fat comes from red animal meats and may be tasty, but should be limited. On the other hand, milk fat is important for your digestion and overall health. It always has been.

Regine Fournier agreed. She's a wonderful example of a traditional French woman – like a perfect baguette, crusty on the outside, warm on the inside. On a recent trip, Dottie and I shared a meal with her and her husband Pierre, a retired fighter pilot hero from the Algerian war who looks exactly like William Shatner.

As a native of south Alabama, I warmed right away the old-South feel of the Maison des Vins in Chalon-sur Saône. The soft colors and wood frame complemented the spacious upstairs veranda. Only the stately oak extending through the floor and ceiling in the corner interrupted the three walls of windows. Regine called it provincial. Not really French, you know, though you might find it off in a colony somewhere.

By the time we got to our cheese course, Regine brought up the issue of the American obsession over fats in the diet. "There are good fats and there are bad fats," she said, brandishing her fork at me with a ripe wedge of St. Marcellin speared on the end. "Duck is fine. Milk fat and olive oil are good. But you have to stay away from pig, sheep, and cow." I asked her how she knew this. I'm American, you know. Show me the data.

I think she enjoyed bouncing back at me that my country "is too young to have a memory." Very matter-of-factly, she told me she knew about healthy fats because her mother had told her, her grandmother had told her mother, and so on. French dietary traditions have been refined, trial and error, for thousands of years. They know it's true because they've already worked it out through the distillation of time. Can't argue with that.

A massive European study called the MONICA project confirms the French intuition on bad fats. It showed that rates of heart disease are 3 times greater for men between the ages of 35 and 64 in Scotland and Ireland than in southern European regions. They certainly don't smoke more than the French, so that's not the cause. But they do eat high quantities of animal tissue fat daily, such as bacon and sausage. Now compare this with the kind of fat eaten by the French.

Boué and his colleagues looked at the fats typically eaten by a large population of healthy French women. Of the "ruminant fats" (which include dairy products, beef, mutton, and tallow), their study showed that the majority of their dietary intake, a full 85% of it, came from dairy products like whole milk and cheeses.

So here's the French recipe for low weight and decreased heart disease: go low on animal tissue fats, high on dairy.

Like the MONICA study, if science knocks around long enough it eventually bumps into the hokey traditions of local common sense and hails them as remarkable discoveries. Recently, it was announced that too little cholesterol can actually *cause* stroke. The oil of walnuts has now been found to *reduce* the risk of heart disease, and an American group found an enzyme in cheese that actually lowers the "bad" cholesterol. In *Eat Fat, Lose Weight*, Dr. Ann Louise Gittleman points out that butter has lecithin (which breaks down bad cholesterol), vitamin A, and the mineral selenium, which is an important antioxidant.

The healthy effects of oils, butters, and other dairy fats only make sense if we look at the world from another angle and begin to see the fat free diet as counterproductive and downright unhealthy. But turning our backs on our assumptions, our deepest beliefs, can be difficult. After all, the daily French baguettes, full fat cheeses (40 – 60% fat), and wine with meals contrasts so sharply with our own experience. We've been riding the low fat train for 30 years now. In spite of this, though, between 1992 and 1999 the number of overweight Americans almost tripled from 34 to 97 million. Unbelievably, over half of the adult population in the U.S. is grossly overweight.

It's ironic to find the highest bulk of overweight people in the same place as you find the largest commitment to diet foods, diet drugs, and economic markets for weight-loss products and programs. How many diet drinks are there? How many low fat, no fat slurries? The conclusion is obvious: all these gimmicks certainly reflect the problem, but have little to do with any effective solution.

That's why it's so astounding that producers keep producing them and consumers keep consuming them. Our economy loves the idea that low fat cuisine is an all-purpose panacea: doing all the good things and avoiding all the bad ones. A million examples stack the shelves, selling us this new pill or that new weight-loss drink. All these products and services represent a 33 billion dollar-per-year industry. 33 billion dollars! All geared toward confirming the dogma that fat is bad, making products and services to combat it, and then telling us how vital it is to buy them.

Perhaps it's not so astounding after all. This self-fulfilling cycle of constant exposure creates a strong aura of authenticity. A case in point is the fat free mantra itself, which is all over books, TV, and radio. With so many people saying the same thing, it must be true. Right?

This fuels the economic pressures behind the huge social dogma that fat is bad – not only for your weight – but for your health too. The result? You'll find no end to the manic search for diets designed to cut the fat, trick it off with brain chemicals, hypnotize it, melt it off with electroshock, or simply suck it out through a tube. All this to make us thin.

That the French ignore our dietary "solutions" is not hard to understand. They don't have a problem. It's stranger that our failure hasn't caused us to look around for approaches that actually work. There's an entire country of people without our problems. We can do what they do.

But have you ever seen children who, when they don't want to hear what someone is telling them, put their fingers in their ears and sing nah, nah, nah, nah, nah, to the tune of "Mary had a little lamb?" When adults indulge in this behavior, it's called the ostrich technique. We could keep on burying our heads in the sand about our weight problems. But it would be more productive to look at the "purple puzzle pieces" of the contradictory French data and try to find out what's wrong with our elaborate, but still very "green" ideas. To begin with, we should start from the more humble premise that we may be more clueless than we think.

Low fat products in your body

When my mom finally returned home from France, she vowed to hold on to the high milk fat diet we had kept up, effortlessly, in France. She must have spent 10 full minutes on the phone with me, ranting about the tiers of no fat/low fat stuff in her Mobile, Alabama grocery store. "It's a big store! Lots of things to buy. But I still can't get anything with a normal amount of fat in it. No wonder these people are so fat!!" She's right, though. Ever look for normal (not low fat) yogurt? You'll burn some calories trying. In the end, mom bought low fat yogurt along with a separate pint of cream. Then she just added it in herself. My mom's feisty.

Pretend for a moment that you have nothing at stake in the question and grant yourself a temporary attitude of skeptical curiosity. Loosely speaking, Americans have all the drugs, all the diet products, and all the fat people. If you have no agenda about this issue other than your own health – if you're not a NutraSweet representative, part of the pharmaceutical industry, or an institutionalized weight-loss clinic – you might say we're missing the boat completely. In looking so hard to find a cheaper, easier way out, we end up overlooking obvious solutions. The result? We ultimately do ourselves a disservice by going so ballistic on one idea – like our fat phobia. Fats, after all, are a normal part of the diet of animals like us. With the help of nutrition and sports physiology research, I want to show how a low fat diet becomes the cause of the problem itself.

To begin with, what happens when you deprive your body of fat? It's well known that fat-deprivation semi-starvation diets lower the metabolic rate, resulting in the body burning less of its energy stores than before. Dr. Wadden and his colleagues have shown that basal metabolic rates can plummet as much as 15% after these types of intense caloric restrictions. Besides the fact that this is not good for you, it effectively retards the point of the diet in the first place. You metabolize energy slower.

But it's even worse than that. The second result is that the body adapts to fat deprivation by *conserving fat*, not burning it (see the chapter "The Science of the French Diet"). Once you return to a normal diet – or, all too commonly, binge – the body's adaptive response preferentially turns the food to fat first. Bottom line: your body needs fat on board, and responds to fat deprivation diets by hoarding fat. It thinks you're starving.

Just as low fat diets decrease the metabolic rate, the opposite is also true. High fat diets increase it. This, by itself, takes the weight off! Back to research. Athletes put on high fat versus low fat diets showed an increase in their body's metabolic rate when eating the higher fat diet. Furthermore, 2 independent labs have shown increases in athlete performance and energy levels (measured as an increase in the time to exhaustion) after only 2 – 4 weeks on a high fat diet. That's why more and more sports nutritionists discourage low fat diets.

Conclusion: once you drop the low fat regime, you have more energy.

Now put these data together.

1) Americans who eat poorly and too much, gain weight.
2) Regardless of the cause, we typically respond by depriving ourselves of food, mainly fat.
3) This insidious strategy lowers our metabolic rate, leaving us with less energy, making us less active, and so making it even harder to get the weight off.
4) Even worse, when we do eat, our body thinks we are starving and so puts on fat first. This leads us to try other diets because our weight keeps growing and growing.

This is the situation we find ourselves in today. Simply put, our body rebels against low fat diets by settling into a negative feedback cycle. How many people do you know who purge themselves on crash diets, loose weight for a week, and then when they do give in and binge, gain it all back again? This type of rubber band effect of weight loss/weight gain is not only unhealthy, but never carries through in the long term. We need an alternative way to think about our diet; one we can apply to our lives for more than a week or month at a time, one that takes off weight without compromising our health.

Searching for home

Rabbit was lost. He had that terrible, sinking feeling. No doubt about it, every time he marched Piglet and Pooh into the mists of the Hundred-Acre Wood, they ended up facing the same sand pit.

He had tried to be clever and strand Tigger in the woods to curtail his socially inappropriate bouncing. But it was Rabbit and his less zealous conspirators who had become confused and lost.

Pooh, however, was led to his larder by a force of gravitation centered about his belly and, in a fit of crystal clear Poohian logic, made the winning suggestion. "Since we walk away from the sand pit looking for home ... and we always end up back at this sand pit ... perhaps when we get out of sight of this sand pit ... well, we should try to find it again. Maybe then we should reach home." Rabbit, frustrated by his inability to complete his dubious plan to discipline Tigger, was in no mood for Pooh's fluff-brained ideas. In the end, though, Rabbit remained lost, bouncily rescued by Tigger. Pooh found home.

Americans, however hard they work at it, keep searching for a way out of their weight problems, and keep ending up back at the same sand pit. But what if one were to take Pooh at his word? What if one were to do what the American system says would make you good and fat, walk away from what we "know" about weight problems, and then try to find it again?

What would it take to design a diet that would be sure to get you back to the sand pit and make you totally fat? First, you would break the cardinal strictures of both schools of dietetic thought: don't avoid fats *or* carbohydrates. For example, you might give yourself full-fat cheeses, whole milk, half-and-half in your coffee, and normal butter (not something with "food product" in the title). Have some empty alcohol calories while you are at it by drinking a touch of wine with your meal. Besides, it goes well with the fresh breads you'll eat for lunch and dinner. Don't be obsessed with exercise; just get out of the house once in a while. Eat late at night and don't have a gigantic breakfast. Maybe take an afternoon nap.

There. The perfect prescription. You'll be big as a house in no time. This, though, as you've probably guessed, is exactly the French diet. The country with an 8% obesity rate! I set up this scenario facetiously, but laughed out loud when I later read the chapter entitled, "The Worst Diet in the World," in a very popular recent diet book. As erudite and confident as Rabbit, the author states that poor health and obesity result from a diet full of "breads and pastries … cheese, butter, cream, and other whole-milk products … [that] get more butterfat into people's systems for good atherogenic measure."

These predictions of gloom and doom, though, fall flat in front of one simple observation: ordinary French people. They're not fat, heart diseased, and their average life span is greater than ours. One clever theory, felled by the plain upright facts.

What the French do right in regard to food and weight doesn't have as much to do with the percent of this or that in their daily intake content of the food web pyramid scheme blabiddy blah, as it does with common sense cultural habits. And you don't have to be afraid of your food or neurotic about calories either. Of course, no one's suggesting you spend all afternoon in a muumuu shoving down cream-filled, fudge-covered Ding Dongs. The prescription of *what* you eat must be balanced with the equally important issue of *when* and *how* you eat. *Diet* isn't so simplistic that you can just sum up the molecular composition of your food. It involves the larger sense of the word – snacking habits, eating routines, and social rules around the table. These suggestions introduce function as well as form, the style of eating as well as the nature of the food.

With this in mind, now we can address the main question. How can the French violate our established dietary rules by eating fats and carbohydrates, without becoming totally fat and unhealthy? The answer, though, is disarmingly simple and do-able. It doesn't emerge from some elegant high-tech Eureka! revelation or miracle cure that melts your fat away with crystals or magnets. It stems from basic rules we've probably all heard growing up. Here are some starters.

Take smaller bites. Don't snack between meals. Finish what you have in your mouth before putting something else in there. Get outside and walk around. Take your time at the table and talk to the people you are eating with. Have some meats, some vegetables, some breads, some desserts – a little of many things is better than a lot of just one. These are simple rules. Very Pooh.

American nutritionists face weight issues like Rabbit: complex and confusing. The French face them more like Pooh:

natural and intuitive. However, despite a thousand Rabbit-like theories, our approach has unfortunately failed to give us any less obesity. In fact, it hasn't even slowed the yearly increases: we can't seem to maintain our current levels of obesity! We try a new diet, circle around again, and find ourselves back at the same sand pit looking for the next hare-brained plan to get us out again.

I believe the solution is simpler than we think. Have you ever rummaged through the fridge for something you knew was there, but just couldn't find? You look behind and under things, rifling through the wilting leftovers in the back, only to find it front row center the whole time – right in front of your nose! The same is true for our diet. After looking so hard for so long, it's time to step back and reconsider what we think we know. First things first.

The Fat Fallacy calls for a clear-headed return to basics. Remember what we have traded in for the impressive complexities of American dietary theories. In two simple components, the French diet takes off weight without even trying. First, don't fear a normal level of fat in your diet (I'll talk about what a "normal" level is in more detail below). Second, adopt eating habits that foster lower weight and a greater appreciation of the food you do eat. In combination, this dietary approach leaves Rabbit's hyper-complexity spinning somewhere out on its own, and takes common sense by the hand on the way to a healthy form for ourselves in the mists.

Faux-Foods Quiz: Kids

Okay, I'll admit it. I'm biased. But let me tell you that I have the 2 coolest children on the planet. There are a billion kids around. And I got the 2 best ones. That's why I feel so lucky.

If you have kids, you know the gratitude you feel for having such wonderful children, despite their foibles, despite the Wild Strawberry and Periwinkle Blue-crayon mural they did to enhance your otherwise boring paint job in the hall. So if you do have children, don't forget to apply these rules to them too. They need the habits of healthy eating to take with them through the rest of their lives. And they also need to eat real food so they can grow up without cavities, allergies, and all the other side effects that come from faux-food additives.

Ingredients

Water, corn syrup, soybean oil, food starch (modified), egg whites, vinegar, salt, maltodextrin, cellulose gum, xanthan gum, carrageenan, natural flavors, color added, mustard flour, sodium benzoate, calcium di-sodium EDTA.

Hint

This is low fat. Therefore, as conventional wisdom tells us, as television ads tell us, as the inertia of our entire American dietary culture tells us, this is good for you. Despite this chatter, the corn syrups, the gums, and all those preservatives make it hard to recognize as a food. If you were to ask Julia Child, she would make this with 5 simple ingredients. All of them can be read by an average second-grader. All of them can be found in a grocery store.

2

A French Love Affair
With Food

Pure attitude.

If we step back far enough, perspective shows us that the differences between French and American eating habits begin with our deepest feelings about our food. Compare our neurotic, even antagonistic, mentality to their *bon vivant* love affair.

Paul Rozin, a scientist who explores the psychology of food, recently surveyed dietary viewpoints from many cultures. He pointed out that the French see food in terms of what it can do for you. Americans, on the other hand, view it in terms of the harm it can inflict: like a pathogen. You look at that slice of pie and see pounds on the scale and saddlebags bulging. You see arteries closing off like collapsing tunnels. Your food nags you to eat more, get fatter, and die of heart disease. What a horrid relationship to have with food.

Unfortunately, this mentality has even insinuated its way into our latest weight loss experts, who offer advice about our food. Barry Sears, for example, author of *The Zone* diet book, was recently quoted as saying that we should view our meal like a drug – some sort of chemical derivative composed of its parts. After reading through the faux-food quizzes, the food manufacturers seem to agree! The French, by contrast, see food as an experience to be enjoyed and the meal as an event to take pleasure in.

Think for a moment about the fear-based, sum-of-the-parts dietary theory. If it were true that the important part of your diet is the bits of ingested food (as some believe), then protein in meat would be just the same as protein in a powder. The nutrient chemicals in a pill would be just the same as those in a balanced meal. This point of view says that it's not important how you get those molecules in your body, just that they get in there. A case in point against this notion is that old theory, now solidly disproved, that a synthesized baby formula is superior to breast milk.

In Dr. Rozin's studies of food attitudes, he asked men and women from several cultures the following question: "If you could satisfy your nutritional needs safely, cheaply and without hunger by taking a daily pill, would you do this?" The starkest contrast in the entire study was between French males (with a resounding No) and American females (who were generally quite happy with this option). The French think pills are for sick people.

Not us. We've come to believe the twisted idea that our food is something bad, something that makes us fat, something that gives us heart disease and diabetes and all the rest. A practical example of this was the almost comic response to a study showing that the beta-carotenes in fruits and vegetables lower your risk of cancer and heart disease. What did we do? Many people might have said, "I see, now I'll eat more fruits and vegetables." Instead it was, "Oh, it must be the beta-carotene that does it. We've found the molecule responsible for good health!"

So pharmaceutical companies cranked up advertisements excited about beta-carotene, millions of Americans swallowed their pills, and it took several years and two major studies to show that eating *synthesized* beta-carotene did nothing whatsoever for your health. 19,939 women took the beta-carotene and 19,937 women took a placebo. Of the women on beta-carotene, 378 got cancer (369 for placebo takers), 42 had heart attacks (50 for placebo takers), and 14 had other cardiovascular-related deaths (12 for the placebo takers). Maybe we should just eat fruits and vegetables. Pills are for sick people.

There's more to our neurotic dietary behavior than just treating our food like a drug, though, because we are also profoundly unhappy about it. To better understand our stomach-grinding worry over foods, Rozin asked other questions like, "Heavy cream belongs best in which category: whipped or unhealthy? Chocolate cake belongs best in which category: guilt or celebration? Ice-cream belongs best in which category: delicious or fattening?"

Americans (guys too, but mainly the women) linked their food to 'unhealthy,' 'guilt,' and 'fattening.' The French related their food to 'whipped,' 'celebration,' and 'delicious.' This love of food is exactly what you observe when you visit France for any length of time.

That's why it was such a shock to come home and notice, as if for the first time, our profound fear and loathing of food. For example, up to 90% of the French answered yes to the following question. "On a vacation, would you choose an average hotel with excellent food over a luxury hotel with average food?" (The price is the same, and you have to eat at the hotel.) As few as 27% of Americans chose the excellent food over shiny elevators and polite bellhops. We insist on exceptional quality in many things. But not in the things we eat.

To see the angst we feel over our food, Rozin made an index to measure issues like "Worry" and "Concern." Unfortunately, the highest ratings fell to the combination of being female and American. Our women go to the greatest lengths to make their diets healthy, and scramble around for all the latest prescribed rules. But even though they try the hardest, they're still the least likely to think they eat healthy food! "Americans seem to have the worst of both worry worlds, the greater concern and the greater dissatisfaction." The French, on the other hand, have the best of both worlds. They have very low worry, very high eating self-esteem, and do not have the health or weight problems that we do.

What's wrong with this picture? Shouldn't being neurotic at least buy us something in return? Unfortunately, it doesn't. We worry about the details, get the least benefit from our frantic uncertainty, and so sweat even more about the details; spinning and spinning into frustrated weight gain and all its associated health problems.

The conclusion of the Rozin study: "We suggest that on the psychological level, Americans may have something to learn from the French." Perhaps what we have to learn from the French is that we need to step away from the old mentality and look at the problem from another perspective. Only in this way can we begin to really change our relationship with our food.

The conclusion of *The Fat Fallacy* is that the French have a way of thinking about their food that brings health, lower weight, and pure pleasure. We should all be able to have this too. By adapting the French dietary habits and foods to the American lifestyle, we can live longer, happier, thinner lives.

Your relationship with your food

We all have relationships: with our parents, children, partners, and coworkers. We have also seen that, for better or worse, we have a relationship with our food. For the French, as we've said, that bond is an *affaire d'amour*. They take their time with this very significant other. They don't hurry through it as if they were too busy with other things. They hold out for the very best. The mature French relationship reinforces important social elements of family and friends, and indulges in the pure sensuality of food.

So where in all our modern dietary advice is the notion of relationship? We typically hear rigorous detail on each variety of protein, fat, and carbohydrate we are allowed, the micronutrients and macronutrients, and the calculated ratio of each. But you won't hear any of that from the French. Their diet veers far and wide of the standard, two-dimensional dietary books, because it encourages us to treat our food like we might a friend (romantic or not). This will make type-A people instantly squeamish and frantic to perform. "Relationship?! How many grams of carbohydrates do I consume before I get to 'relationship'?" But as I'll show, this idea is natural and intuitive, and applies just as well for your spouse, partner, or friend.

Begin with the most obvious rule of all. Take your time. Don't rush it. Have you ever been in a conversation with someone and felt like you were just something they had to do on the way to something else? A healthy relationship with your food begins by paying attention to what you eat. All too often, the joy of eating becomes the mechanics of ingestion when the meal gets set on the brain's back burner

> **Enjoyment and satisfaction have more to do with the amount of time you spend on the meal than the raw poundage of food you consume.**

while watching re-runs, driving, or walking back to the office.

This simple beginning accomplishes several things at once. You begin to eat smaller bites, making quality more important than quantity, and enjoying what you eat even more. The word "savor," for example, has no meaning at all if you gulp everything so fast that you never even taste it.

Just think about the basics of eating. Taste buds are on your tongue. You've seen people who take such gargantuan bites that their mouth brims with food and their cheek is packed solid. They can't even taste the majority of the food they're swallowing whole. They're doing something. But, whatever it is, it's not about tasting the food.

A healthy relationship with your food allows you to appreciate eating at a relaxed pace that benefits you. Fortunately, you are more in control of this kind of relationship than most others. Unlike your partner, you can determine exactly what all facets of this significant other – your food – is like. As opposed to personal relationships, where each of you can have competing agendas, foibles, and weaknesses to work through, developing a relationship with your food is completely under your control. Also, there's no problem leaving one set of foods for another.

Think about it like sex. When you're young, you can't wait to *do it*. Then when it does happen, 4.75 frenzied seconds later, it's over. Girls with Harlequin romance visions say, "That's it?" Guys, on the other hand, say, "That was great!" In fact, the whole point for the immature guy is the climax itself – the very thing that means it's over! It's the product, not the process. Americans rush to the end of a meal like the frantic tryst of a ravenous 19-year-old.

It's not just the time taken, either. Quality gets a backseat too. For the immature guy, as the saying goes, there is no bad sex. You can have the thin veneer of beauty make-upped over the top – or not. And food can have a clever wrapper plastered with an artsy photograph – or not. Those are irrelevant details.

> ### Key principles of
> ### *The Fat Fallacy*
>
> 1. **Eating habits develop your relationship with your food.**
> 2. **A bad relationship will make you fat.**

From a dietary standpoint, Americans go for the quickie. The point of eating is to finish. Finish and then do something else. Thus, *the process of eating* becomes nothing more than the interval before we've satisfied our urge and we can go back to "important" things. You can see how the French view American fast food as a type of culinary prostitution.

Somehow we've come to this twisted conclusion: if you love your food, you have to eat it as if you've been starving your whole life. You have take huge bites. Gulp it down. "Man," we say, "look how fast I finished all that." Enjoying your food means getting to the end as fast as you can. It means spending as little time eating as possible! Does that make sense?

This way of relating to our food needs to be changed. We need to think differently and approach diet and health from a mature point of view. This implies, of course, that we've been holding immature points of view, but these can be "up-graded" very easily if we want them to be.

In the end, this is about you. What kind of relationship do you want to have? Is your goal just to finish and then roll off to something else? Or do you want a relationship where you take your time, where the point is to savor the process, where you want to enjoy it as long as possible?

Such a healthy relationship requires some commitment to retraining how we think – buying quality food, allotting the time to enjoy the process of eating, and making eating a social affair. The meal is something to seek out, not treat like a nuisance. Food is a pleasure, not something to be inhaled so quickly you can't even taste it. Retraining what and how we eat ultimately builds this new relationship. Some will undoubtedly see it as ironic that, in the end, simply interacting in a healthy way with your food is all that's needed to take the weight off.

Quality, not quantity

Our normal dietary knee-jerk response tells us to micromanage our diet. How many grams? How many slices? Is this an empty calorie? What's my glycemic index? We all want to be methodical and rigorous, and do whatever we have to do to lose the weight. In this way, though the effort is well intentioned, we end up looking too closely at the bits and overlooking the big picture. We're overloaded with trees, and don't get nearly enough of the forest.

Over the past 25 years, scientists have provided us with steady argumentation about which major nutrient needs to be factored out of our diet: carbohydrates, fats, or proteins. These debates go on and on. In the most recent high-profile event, the USDA gathered together a "summit" of diet gurus. They all described their plans, and squabbled over who got to claim which scientific evidence for their nutrient to be the critical one.

Much of this confusion appears because of the way we've chosen to look at the problem in the first place. We generally think of food as bits of data entered into our body's computer, and blow off the context in which it is eaten. In my view, a crucial next step for nutritional research will be outside this well-worn box. We need to consider more than just the molecules. Context matters!

Here is an example that makes the point. Even if you eat low fat foods, but eat them in a great hurry, you end up eating more food and gaining weight. The flip side is also true. Even if you increase your fat intake, but eat it slower, you end up eating less overall and losing weight. I go into this in detail in the chapter, "The Plan: How We Should Eat."

An essential message of *The Fat Fallacy* is that eating richer quality foods leaves you more satisfied with less food. And the effects of eating less quantity are stunning, as long as you have a balanced diet of real foods. Dr. Leakey and his colleagues (in the *International Journal of Toxicology*) reported a list of health benefits from decreasing your food intake, including increased life span and metabolic efficiency. This is in addition to the decreased rates of cancer, cardiovascular disease, and diabetes. These are brilliant effects. And all *you* have to do is eat delicious food, and focus on savoring every bite.

If a pharmaceutical company had invented a pill that did all this, it would be hailed as a miracle drug and pushed through the FDA approval process with an extruder. But the French dietary habits can't be patented. It's hard to cut a profit on good sense alone.

One more incredible finding by Dr. Duffy and his colleagues multiplies the effect of eating rich, high quality foods (see Appendix: "Diet and the Metabolic Rate"). Experimental animals that weren't allowed to stuff themselves actually changed their eating habits! "A change was also observed in feeding behavior, with shifts away from a snacking pattern toward a meal pattern. As caloric intake decreased, ... they became more like meal feeders and less likely to nibble." Who wouldn't like this to happen to them or their children? Translation: the more you eat, the more you want to eat.

More importantly, getting off low fat diets decreases your likelihood of getting cancer. In a recent article in *Toxicological Sciences*, Walter Willett pointed out that high fat diets lowered the chances of getting cancerous tumors. But this only happened when the total amount of food decreased. You still can't gorge on it like a frenzied hyena on the savannas ripping apart your latest downed antelope. You must take smaller bites and savor your food.

The Fat Fallacy diet provides a way to eat as much wonderful food as you are hungry for. You stop eating when you are pleasantly satisfied. The key to keep from going overboard is to follow the habits of healthy eating listed here. This effectively enlists your body's natural physiological responses to get you there. More importantly, the rules I advise make complete intuitive sense, no mental gymnastics required.

French and American eating habits

I know I'm in America. But I'm going to commit a serious heresy – on purpose. I realize that there is no way to market habits in pill-form, but I'm going to throw it out there anyway: your health and your weight don't just depend on *what you eat*, but also *how you eat*. In this section, I hope to convince you that your eating habits have a larger influence on your weight than the latest dietary gimmick: calorie counter, weight index calculator, weight-loss pill, fat free candy, diet soft drink, or passive electrolytic fat burner! In this diet, you don't need to buy anything. Just embrace the habits of healthy eating.

First, let's look at the standard habits we're working with.

A colleague in France told me that he went to see a movie while visiting friends here in the U.S. He was incredulous at how many people could not sit through one film without getting up in the middle and going to get another tub of popcorn and a drink. "Maybe," he said, "they're so used to commercials on TV, where they can get up and browse the refrigerator, that they have to do it at the movies too." He found it bothersome to try to watch the movie with everyone getting up and sitting down all the time.

I went to the movies on several occasions while I lived in France. The cinema staff always came into the theater just before the film started. The person working the concessions carried in a cardboard box full of about 6 different kinds of candies and ice creams. Everyone swarmed the guy in a sort of mass action semi-circle. When they'd gotten what they wanted, he whipped the remainders into his impromptu carrier and took it all away, into the dim back room, never to return. We were expected to watch the movie. They must figure that if you can't make it though a two-hour film that's supposed to divert your attention anyway, you should see a doctor, not a movie.

Have you noticed that Americans graze all the time? We nibble away on mounds of snacky chips, cookies, and stuff of every imaginable consistency and shade of neon. I didn't really notice this until I came back home, stunned by some very common things – like the ends of grocery aisles. They're completely different in the U.S. and France.

In France, you typically find coffee here, toilet paper there, wine on the end of this aisle, and canned fish beside those little dry biscuits on another. But go into any U.S. supermarket. Chips in bags are at the end of aisle 1, sweets stacked on soft drinks on aisles 2 – 4, chips in cans as you turn out of aisle 5, the Keebler elf and his assortment of fat free cookies as you approach the canned soup section, and an assortment of weight-loss slurries at the end of the aisle devoted to junk food.

Our preoccupation with snacks helps explain the most obvious difference between the habits of these two cultures. Americans snack all the time, whereas the French eat at meal times.

Making it last

Other French eating habits are well known. First of all, breakfast is small. They're basically a night-loving people who get up late and stay up late – not the chipper, happy-in-the-morning crowd. By the time they roll out of bed, it's getting close to lunch anyway. But they are most famous for the luxurious length of their meals. At lunches and dinners, it's common to eat, sip, and talk for two hours or more. As your basic American in France, it was hard to imagine taking so long to eat.

The Reader Replies: Kim and Alex

Just wanted to drop you a note to let you know that things are going quite well for Alex and me. We started Saturday the 6th, and are sailing along. I can already eat just at mealtimes. What's incredible, however, is that I'm full and satisfied on so much less food, and I'm actually enjoying my meals much more. Needless to say, we're having a ton of fun on it, getting more satisfaction from less food. As an added bonus, I've lost 3 lbs this first week! (Alex is very tall and thin, and could actually stand to gain some weight, so hopefully I'll lose and he'll stay the same!)

Warmest Regards, Kim and Alex

I just wanted to give you an update – Alex and I hit our "week 8" last weekend. We each got on the scale, and I'm down a total of 8 pounds! Alex has also lost 5 pounds – which is weight he really didn't need to lose, but he looks great! I'm down 1-2 sizes (depending on the designer), and Alex is fitting into pants he wore in college. Most importantly, however, we feel great!

Thanks, again, for the book! You really have helped to improve our lives, and our waistlines!

Kim

But embracing healthy French eating habits is critical, because increasing your food quality only decreases the quantity if you take your time. This is why so many studies on weight gain and high fat diets are hard to interpret – they don't control for how fast or slow people eat. If two groups eat the very same food – but one gulps it down and the other eats it slow – the 2nd group will give themselves time to feel full, snack less between meals, and lose more weight. How you eat is important!

This fact resolves a "mystery" of nutrition science. How can the French people eat what they do, and not become overweight and heart diseased like us? One reason is that, by ignoring the eating rate, we end up probing a 3-dimensional problem with only 2-dimensional tests. This leaves us very confused by the answers we find. It's like trying to figure out what a cat is by holding it high over your head and only looking down at its flat shadow on the ground. You can turn it over and around, but a flat image of a round object is very difficult to resolve.

Once we factor in the French eating habits, more of the dietary picture begins to take shape in front of us.

1. Basic social rules of the meal encourage you to eat slower.
2. Eating slower allows your body to let you know you are full before you overeat.
3. Eating less food makes you lose weight.

It's a very simple idea.

So lets look at the length of the French meal. Are they given more food among their several courses, therefore taking longer to eat it? Or, since they encourage conversation with family and friends over the meal, you might think it lasts longer due to the distraction of talking all the time. Or, given the savory nature of the food, perhaps they take longer to enjoy each bite. The answer lies in their ingrained cultural rules of eating.

There are many of these rules, but we can distill out two very important aspects of the meal. First, no one starts eating until everyone has their food and all can be wished a "*bon appetit.*" Second, the next course of food is never put on the table until the first one is done.

Even if one person finishes the first course, the next portion isn't brought out until everyone at the table has finished. Only then, after some delay, does the main course come out so everyone can begin eating again. *Bon appetit.* The same is true for the cheese course and finally the dessert. Waiting for everyone to finish encourages an extended, enjoyable social atmosphere around eating. A "meal," then, isn't just the food. The meal is a social gathering that includes food. The point is not to get full. The point is to be together.

Separating the courses and having the manners to wait to eat until everyone has their food, naturally makes the meal take a long time. More importantly, this leaves you feeling satisfied but never overly stuffed. Actually, I only felt bloated-full once during my entire stay in France. We prepared a traditional Thanksgiving meal for my boss and his family, complete with mashed potatoes and turkey and gravy and peas and pickles and sweet potatoes and cranberry sauce. It was painful. I was stuffed.

There's no French equivalent for the phrase "pig out," or the American tendency to wolf down their food. If you had to pinpoint this difference, you would say that the French eat, Americans feed. Once you notice this ravenous "feeding" behavior, you begin to see it everywhere. When the food arrives, everything becomes absolutely silent. On your mark. Get set. Eat! Then faces are full until some decide to come up for air.

Restaurants reinforce this unfortunate habit. Ever been to a Chinese restaurant and, before your hot and sour soup gets cool enough to eat, the Hunan shrimp is plunked down right beside it? This is particularly annoying because you have to choke back the first course so the second isn't stone cold by the time you get to it. To have a greater customer flow rate, they want patrons to get in and get out. Waiters make tips by the table and hustle to get more people through in a night. Your bill (to pay when you leave) is often given to you as soon as your food arrives.

In French restaurants, customers don't have to tack on an additional tip. Although this does help create the famous "attitude" of French waiters, they don't need to shove you out the door or ask you repeatedly if there's anything else you need before you leave.

We're left with a regrettable comparison of our cultures. For us, eating is a hurried and incidental via point between errands. For them, it's a luxurious commitment to enjoyment, not a distracting means to some other end. Eating is for pleasure. It is the end itself.

Faux-Foods Quiz: Stealth food products

Go to the grocery store. If you see a 5-lb bag of titanium di-oxide on the shelf, please send me an email and let me know. I went to an air show once to see the newest, fastest jets on the planet. The announcer told us that one of them was reinforced with titanium something. Why is this jet component on a food ingredient list? Don't do an Internet search for titanium di-oxide. It's scary.

The same thing is true for calcium silicate, which sounds like it might be a component of Formica, concrete, or plaster. The truth isn't much better. Actually it's used for insulation applications in power plants, chemical plants, shipyards, refineries, and paper mills. Magnesium oxide? I don't want that touching my skin.

The only real redeeming factor of the concoction below is that its two main ingredients are sugar and fructose. If you sweeten the hell out of magnesium oxide, calcium silicate, and titanium di-oxide, at least it tastes pretty good.

Ingredients
Sugar, fructose, citric acid, magnesium oxide, natural flavor, calcium silicate, lemon juice solids, ascorbic acid, titanium di-oxide, yellow 5 lake, artificial flavor, BHT.

Hint
This thing provides the greatest contrast between something that should be simple and wholesome, and something that's an amazing accumulation of chemicals. Go with the original version. It tastes great and it's better for you.

SOCIAL, POLITICAL, & NUTRITIONAL SCIENCE

3

When Science
Looks in the Mirror

Objective interpretation is an oxymoron.
The reason for this is that scientists are human beings, not
computers. They have as many preconceived notions and gut
feelings to guide them as anyone else. These normal scientific
biases come in two flavors. One of them is natural, unavoidable,
and unconscious. The other involves uglier conflicts of interest.
Let's look at the first case, where someone's simple assumptions
about the world end up leaving a few results highlighted and the
rest completely ignored.

We can start with a bit of science: a "correlation
analysis." A correlation analysis is done when you want to know
if two things are related (like fat intake and weight gain). You
just look to see if **A** changes when **B** does. If **A** goes up and **B**

goes up too, they may be related (there's a logical flaw – a fly in the soup – but I'll get to that below).

Let's say we want to know the effect of fat consumption (**A**) on obesity rates (**B**). First we would check to see whether their changes mirror each other. Now what do the data say? As for fat intake, a Harvard study found that Americans reduced their saturated fat intake from 15.58% in 1980 to only 10.63% in 1990, indicating a steady decline over 10 years. Over the past 30 years, Americans have decreased total fat consumption by 15%. This is what they told us to do. This is what we did.

So that's **A**. As for **B**, the National Heart, Lung, and Blood Institute estimated that almost twice as many Americans are obese now compared to 1960 (an increase from 13% to 22.5%). The most recent estimates put that rate at a whopping 33%. In the U.S., well over half of the population is grossly overweight, Biggie-sized. The fact that childhood obesity has now blipped onto the nation's health radar is something we should be ashamed of. Weight-related problems kill 300,000 Americans every year. From 1980 to 1990, incidences of both heart disease and obesity have gone up, not down. That's **B**.

Fat consumption fell, obesity rates rose. That's odd. Not what we thought would happen at all. We expected our national experiment in fat free eating to show us that if we did what they said to do, we'd get thinner. But the message is exactly the opposite. Eat less fat, get more obese.

Ah hah! There's the fly in the correlation soup! Just because two things go up or down together doesn't mean they're related. There may be other factors involved. What about exercise? We must be less active now. That would explain why *decreasing* fat consumption is correlated with *increasing* weight problems.

But the "fitness revolution" started in the 1970's and continued through the 1980's. And as pointed out before, activity levels from 1991 to 1998 generally increased. Americans were told that being more active is good for you, and we did what they said. Unfortunately, though, an increase in exercise alone was not enough to overcome our mounting weight problems when we kept to the yellow-brick fat free road.

Dr. Steven Blair is a fitness researcher at the Cooper Institute in Dallas, Texas. He adhered to the American Heart Association's low fat recommendations religiously. He ran 30 miles a week. If anyone on the planet should be able to lose weight – or at the very least, maintain weight, it should be this man. But even with his low fat diet, *despite his high level of physical activity*, he still reported in the *New York Times* that he gradually packed on 25 extra pounds over a few years!

Now what? Increasing weight problems correlate with a low fat diet, even in the face of the benefits of exercising more. Eat low fat and exercise and still gain weight. This never made the front-page news: no press conference, no cameras, no revelations. Maybe it's that fly again, or maybe we're on the wrong page altogether.

A more subtle and important reason this strong result didn't appear throughout the news media is that we don't really believe it to begin with. Even though it comes from very carefully controlled studies, the results disagree with what we expected to find before we looked at the data in the first place. Imagine how different it would have been if the study had concluded that "exercise and low fat diets make you thin and healthy." We would have heard all about these exciting results, because that's what everyone predicted from the beginning.

Of course, no one would say, "I'm going to do this study. But if I find results I don't like, I'll just look the other away and do another study that gives me 'better' results." No one says that. But that's what happens.

Why? If you do a huge study, using a ton of government grant money, and get results that don't make sense (like the low fat/weight gain example), you have two choices. First, you could assume that the study was flawed somehow: instrument failure, method failure, phase of the moon is off, experimenter failure. There could be any number of flies buzzing around in there somewhere that messed up the results you knew you should have gotten.

Otherwise, you have to assume that the data are correct and all your ideas and beliefs are wrong. This means that you're thinking about it all wrong, and now you have to reorient everything you've ever said in public about fat and weight. Scientists, like anyone else, will disbelieve a study's experimental methods, designs, and details, long before they'll throw away their gut feelings and deepest beliefs.

That's the problem. Our data need to agree with what we already believe. If you planted a seed you knew was a tomato, and two weeks later a tomato came up you'd say, "Ah hah ... tomatoes ... I knew it!" Time for a press conference.

On the other hand, if a carrot popped up instead, you'd say, "Who put that carrot here?" When the results deviate from what we expect, we have no way to explain them. You can't even talk intelligently about these results. That's only natural. What would you say, anyway? "My, well ... that's weird ... now what?" Nobody wants to hear that.

Look at the flip side. Imagine what would happen if we did the same experiment, got the same results, but this time had the opposite beliefs going into it. What if we "knew" that a reasonable level of fat in our diets *prevented* heart disease and weight gain? We would

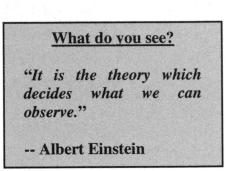

What do you see?

"It is the theory which decides what we can observe."

-- Albert Einstein

look at all the people who have been on low fat diets these past 30 – 40 years and we'd see that we've got enormous weight and heart problems as a result. "Ah hah ... I knew it! Tomatoes!!"

We'd hold up the French diet as a model we should follow, and puzzle over why anyone would adopt a low fat lifestyle. Instead we do exactly the reverse. Here's the point: our culture has expectations, and scientists are no less human than anyone else. This fixes the scientific mindset of the day on its dogma when looking at the data. Seek and ye shall find.

Faith in science

Science has a parental air of authority. It bestows new facts and figures about the world as we look on, clearly impressed. Who can argue with the stunning progress we've made in curing diseases and making our lives easier on a daily basis? Science says X and we answer, "Yes sir. Thank you sir."

But what about nutritional science? From the public's point of view, they seem to bicker and waffle over new conflicts each year. What happened? These scientists are just as brilliant as any others, and clearly expend a lot of effort uncovering the mysteries of the body in relation to food. All their work, though, hasn't deflated our swelling crisis of confidence in them.

Remember when all oils were bad for you? Some researchers still believe this, even today. But, for the time being, we now hear that olive oil plays an important preventative role in heart disease. Remember when eggs were so bad for you that the lab coats on your television baritoned their warnings about the cholesterol time bomb that will make you fat and kill you? At the time, people said, "Eggs? Aren't eggs good for you? It's an egg." But they deferred to science because scientific research must know something they don't. Look at all their data, charts, curving lines, and that very impressive vocabulary.

Boomerang. Now there's another study showing that even though eggs have loads of cholesterol (a whopping 215 milligrams in a large one), diabetics aside, it does not make people more likely to have heart problems at all! A Harvard Study published in the *Journal of the American Medical Association* determined that about an egg per day on average causes no harm whatsoever. More lab coats, more data, more vocabulary. Now you can eat eggs.

But nutrition science consistently stuck to its guns, urging us to give up as many fats as we can. They leaned on lab rat research and population studies showing that high fat diets caused breast cancer. This conclusion was gospel until a massive 14-year study on almost 90,000 women (ages 30 – 55, completed in March of 1999) showed no relation whatsoever between high fat diets and breast cancer (another *JAMA* study).

Now high fat diets have nothing to do with a woman's chance of getting breast cancer. Even worse, low fat diets did not protect them from it either. In fact, women who ate the least fat were the most likely to get breast cancer (15% greater risk!). Most surprisingly, it didn't even matter whether these women had the "good" kind or the "bad" kind of fat. These results make absolutely no sense to the dogged mentality of fat free eating.

But we plod on; still recommending the fat free diet, hoping our data will begin to make sense. The scientific inertia behind our cultural fat phobia, however, has finally started to sputter. After all the work on fats as a health hazard, Dr. Gerald Reaven, professor of medicine at Stanford University, broke from the pack. After more than 20 years studying heart disease, he has decided that the real problem isn't fat or cholesterol at all, but a more integrative problem with the body's alchemy: particularly insulin. His book on "Syndrome X" stressed that we should have more foods with fat, not less.

We can talk about good fats and bad fats later, but first let's get the skeletons out of the closet. The old fat free diet doesn't work, and Reaven shows that it can even be deadly.

As you might imagine, with everyone sticking to their guns, there is huge disagreement out there. Compare Reaven's conclusions to those of Dr. Dean Ornish, who tells people in his Sausalito California Preventive Medicine Institute to do precisely the opposite. Limit your fat consumption to only 10% of your total intake. 10%! That's what Reaven and the *JAMA* study say will kill you.

Now hear Dr. Atkins tell you how important it is for you to avoid carbohydrates like the plague. But the International Food Information Council hates this diet. They say his plan causes ketosis, which causes nausea, dehydration, dizziness, headaches, and diarrhea. Great.

Talk to one doctor and you get one story with loads of data and vocabulary. Talk to another doctor and you get another story with another set of data – same vocabulary. Eggs, no eggs; fat, no fat; carbs, no carbs. You say po-Tay-toe, I say po-Tah-toe, lets call the whole thing off. No wonder people treat what they hear with a grain of salt. It seems that the only consistent fact is that the reports change faster than scenes in an MTV video.

I don't want to create the sense that dietary research science is somehow bogus, because it's not. They contend with two fundamental problems. The first comes from the fact that their scientific community is in a sort of crisis mode, like playground kids winging pebbles at each other. This happens when the standard way of thinking no longer works, agreement dissolves, and medical clinics divide in dramatic debates over which facts are even relevant! Think about the students that come out of each of these schools. They will "grow up" to be unfamiliar with the other's assumptions and methods and procedures – against them from the start. That's why they talk past each other much of the time.

The other very real problem *is not science*, but our *image of science*. All those scientists and their data and jargon come to us pre-packaged from TV and newspaper media – whose aim is to sell you a story. Science, schmience, there's ratings to be had.

A recent article about science and the media addressed this problem head on. It asked whether scientific progress on diet was helped or hurt by highly publicized findings from single studies. This article reported what we all know. Five years ago, a full "78% of primary household shoppers believed it 'very likely' or 'somewhat likely' that in the next 5 years experts would have a completely different idea about which foods were healthy and which were not." As we've seen, the respondents in the survey were absolutely right. First you hear one thing, then you hear another. Nutrition science says X, and we answer "Right. Yaddie Yadda."

For their part, research clinics need to get their results out of sterile academia and into the real world. And who, really, is going to curl up with the latest issue of a dietary science journal? Nobody. To reach the world, then, science ends up in a necessary dance with the devil. Sure, the media can be powerful allies to reach the masses in the short term, but can also be ultimately harmful in the long term because these channels have their own agendas. This is where our image of science gets messed up. Why? Because science is "evolutionary, not revolutionary." It takes time to build up enough evidence to be sure that the data mean what we think they mean.

Scientists are generally skeptical people who read a study critically and try to find any of the thousand reasons the results could be misleading and wrong. Even if the work was done well enough so there aren't obvious fatal flaws, the data could still be biased in some other unforeseen way.

We scientists are trained in graduate school to ferret out those errors. Major kudos go to the student who can point out the critical error that makes a paper meaningless. Mambo brownie points there.

Particularly in areas of dramatic uncertainty, like diet, a scientific result must percolate up in status – from garbage to possible to probable – over years of confirmation. Data aren't innocent until proven guilty, they are suspect until proven and proven and proven reliable. This means

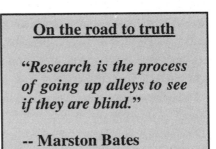

On the road to truth

"Research is the process of going up alleys to see if they are blind."

-- Marston Bates

that conclusions aren't birthed from the test tube of a single study. When scientists appear on the screen with "the hottest new finding," it may be catchy in the media, but not on the front lines of research. It has to be replicated in many different conditions by people who are inherently skeptical in the first place. This, however, would be a bit blasé for the nightly newsflash. Dr. Greenwald stated it best in the *Journal of Nutrition*: "although reports in the popular press frequently tout one food or another as the 'cure for cancer,' nutritional scientists long ago rejected such claims."

Now you see the problem. One hot newsworthy study doesn't mean much until it's been repeated so many times that it's no longer a hot newsworthy study. And the doctor on the latest front-page story seems like the boy who cried wolf when the headlines treat preliminary findings as final conclusions, rather than the questionable pieces of a puzzle that may be tossed out tomorrow. This is how the *presentation of science*, not science itself, sours people to the latest research results.

Here's a specific example from nutrition science.

Remember the headline: "Low fat diets decrease the bad cholesterol that leads to heart disease." This news release leads us to believe that low fat diets are the super-highway to health, happiness, and smaller pants. But scientists know that these diets not only lower LDL, but also the protective cholesterol, HDL. This messy detail makes it more complicated. If they told you both of these facts, you would wonder how losing your protective HDL balanced out with also losing the harmful LDL. Is more of the good stuff lost than bad stuff, or vice versa? Off camera, scientists throw up their hands and get back to work sorting this out. So what you hear from the screen and what happens in the lab, are often two different things.

Just to set this last point straight, the ratio of HDL to LDL is another one of those issues that are still unresolved. One research group thinks it's more beneficial to be low fat and lower the LDLs. Others say that high fat diets "may be preferable to a low fat diet because of more favorable effects on the cardiovascular disease risk profile." How it balances out was stated best in a scientific journal, not on the nightly news. "The overall risk is based on inter-individual differences in response to these nutrients." (Don't worry, I speak scientist. He said that everybody's different so you can't really tell.) This means it's not ironed out yet, or very sellable either.

Uncertainty is rarely newsworthy, and media stories need absolute values, not messy data. Unfortunately, we live in a messy world, and science is a messy business. So, when the lab coats on the news report reverse themselves, again, it drives home the skepticism.

This is why the honeymoon of nutrition science and the public is over. The result, though, might not be so bad. On one hand, you could look at it and think that Americans are becoming more cynical of what they see and hear. But maybe this cynicism is better described as savvy. Perhaps we're simply becoming as dubious of upstart scientific results as scientists are themselves. That's fair enough.

Political science, social science

I hope you're coming to a healthy skepticism of single-shot scientific studies that appear in the news. Another reason to be wary of what you read – even of the official word from Washington – has to do with the second unfortunate problem of conflict of interests. The Physicians Committee for Responsible Medicine recently went to court, and sued the Departments of Agriculture and Health and Human Services because six out of the eleven members who created our National Dietary Guidelines have ties to various beef and dairy industries. The Dietary Guidelines form the template for federal food programs like the School Lunch Program, the School Breakfast Program, and the Food Stamp Program.

When this story went public, Nicholas Regush, a medical columnist for ABC News, responded that "it wouldn't surprise me in the least if I suddenly learned that all the members of the government committee that recommends national health policy were in bed with one industry or another. I wouldn't even blink." Their conclusions are just as objective as the tobacco industry researchers who, with very sincere faces, wave around data telling us that cigarettes are neither addictive nor lethal.

Given the number of committee members linked to the beef and dairy industries, their recommendations not surprisingly emphasize the consumption of meat and dairy products. In fact, the lawsuit suggests that our government's official Dietary Guidelines read more like an ad campaign for these industries than a balanced set of dietary rules. Other associations see this public relations gravy train and bang at the door to get their people on the panel. Is there no place to get unbiased advice?

Of course, you can crack open any nutritionist journal (where they have to list their funding sources) and dig around for scientists who are not getting paid by some food industry. But this requires that you wade through an impenetrable jargon swamp of methods, results, and materials. Even worse, if you make it this far you'll find dietary advice sprawling off like kudzu vines in summer.

This confusing lack of agreement only means that legitimate scientists are exploring the unstable boundary of what we know. Out there at the edge, false starts and hopeful tries often fall through and have to be restarted from scratch. They're approaching a very difficult problem. It'll take some time to sort it all out.

In the meantime, don't believe everything you hear.

Conflict of interest: A case in point

The Canadian Sugar Institute (CSI) is an association of sugar manufacturers. They produce scientific information for health professionals, educators, and the media to promote sugar in diet. They make it, and they want people to buy it.

It's not surprising, then, to hear their lobby state that there "are no data to suggest that consumers should limit the amount of sugars or other types of carbohydrates they eat." This is straight from Dr. Harvey Anderson, Professor of Nutritional Sciences and Physiology, University of Toronto (a member, I might add, of the Canadian Sugar Institute Nutrition Advisory Panel).

If a judge were to rule on a case involving sugar, and that judge had a major financial interest in the sugar industry, we'd call him biased and his judgments flawed. It's standard procedure for those people to recuse themselves. It's surprising how this same logic doesn't get applied to scientists.

(Source: http://www.sugar.ca/USDAresp.htm)

Who's leading this dance?

This brings me to another irony of science and the public. Laboratory science does not always lead us – as they do when, for example, they discover something and we all say, "Ahh" and then make that discovery a part of our lives (like the polio vaccine). Nutrition science is the perfect example of the other side of the coin, when simple observations lead science along new paths.

Research laboratories did not do thousands of tests and come to the logical conclusion that olive oil was good for you and reduced your risk of heart disease. Rather, it resulted when we noticed that people in countries like Spain and France are very healthy. "They don't have as much heart disease. They're not huge. Neat." Only now do we begin the process of finding out *why this is true*. It turns out that olive oil may be a big factor in this healthy equation. In this case, ordinary experience and observations lead science forward.

Anyone who's ever been to the Mediterranean can tell you that their diet is beneficial psychologically and physically. The scientific why and wherefore will follow soon enough. In the meantime, why shouldn't we just do what they do?

As in the olive oil example, science will eventually come around to tell us what we already know and can plainly see – that (non-animal tissue) fat is good for you, that you should eat smaller portions, that wine is good for you, that moderation will save your life, etc. We'll read the report in all its wordy details and extended references at the end. But today, we'll have to trust our observations about what works, what doesn't, and then follow those leads.

I'll get little resistance when I use the example of olive oil to make this point. But I expect to trigger the "fight or flight" response when I use the same logic for cheese and dairy products. Cheese is an embarrassing stepchild to nutrition research. Just listen to the old school scientists trying to explain the benefits of the Mediterranean diet. They completely avoid mentioning the fact that the French eat tons of silky crumbly yummy cheeses with every meal but breakfast. This drives them crazy! For

American nutritionists, the cheese factor is a great big bloody rhinoceros head right in the middle of the floor during a dinner party. No one mentions it, and everyone talks around it as if it weren't there.

It just makes no sense to our current dogma. So you hear some researchers go on and on about the intake of omega-3 fatty acids found in fish – very trendy right now. These are indeed important, but the French eat a lot more full fat cheeses than they do fish. Silence. Maybe if we ignore it, it'll go away. "What rhinoceros head? I don't see any rhinoceros head." But in 5 more years studies will come out telling us what we plainly see from the Mediterranean diet: full fat cheeses in moderation are part of a diet that is healthy for your weight and heart.

Now do one more correlation analysis. High fat dairy foods, high carbohydrate breads, and wine are ubiquitous parts of the French diet, but not the American diet. They have low rates of obesity and heart disease. **That's A.** The American research culture believes in their heart of hearts that fat levels in a normal French diet are harmful. **That's B.** Even though the French diet provides plenty of valid scientific data, our cultural assumptions make us either stammer to explain it or ignore it altogether. If we were writing about science itself, we might say that our scientific conclusions correlate better to our cultural beliefs than our results.

Just a thought.

The Reader Replies: Carrie

I understand what you mean (I'm beginning to ...) about having a relationship w/ your food. We're loving the food. I can't tell you how much fun I've had planning, shopping and cooking. I'm already a really good cook, but I've been able to ratchet it up another notch. I feel free-er to choose full fat foods that everyone knows are more fun to cook and serve. We have a *fabulous* market down the street from our house. I go shopping w/ a short list of staples and then let the food talk to me. Since I'm only buying for two meals, I can plan on the spot in the market w/o overindulging my budget or time. I'm babbling . . . but you can tell that I love food.

We're also eating in courses, we got rid of the crap in our refrigerator (my husband, miracles of miracles, gave up the M&M's voluntarily), we have good snacks on hand (5 different cheeses, crackers, olives, fruit, fresh veggies, and whole milk yogurt), and we have red wine in the rack. Life is good.

It took about one week to get the portion size down. Even in this short period of time it looks vulgar to eat such huge quantities or to eat in the car or to gulp my food at my desk. I discovered that I never chewed my food. Just making that change is huge. I love the personal strategies that you recommend. I put my fork down between bites. It works beautifully. And feels more civilized.

I'm very grateful for your book.

Talk to you soon.
C.

Faux-Foods Quiz: Paints, plastics, and glues. Oh my!

The thing to notice about this very common product is that, before sodium caseinate (whatever that is), it's pretty much just a sugar and partially hydrogenated soybean oil slurry. Notice that ingredients show up on the list by quantity, so whichever one makes up the greatest proportion goes first.

Ingredients
Sugar, partially hydrogenated soybean oil, corn syrup solids, sodium caseinate, di-potassium phosphate, mono and di-glycerides, soy lecithin, decaffeinated instant coffee, natural and artificial flavors, sodium citrate.

Hint
This faux-food tastes good. No doubt about that. And the ads really draw you in and make you want to be that person on the screen. That's why so many people love Victoria Secret magazines. If you just had that product, then you would poke out of your clothes just like that, your lips would pout, and rock stars would be climbing all over you.

But you don't have to keep a quart of partially hydrogenated soybean oil on your shelf to get this product, or pretend you are that snuggly person on the screen, curled up on the couch with a good book.

By the way, I looked up "casein" just to see what it was. This is straight out of the dictionary. "A white, tasteless, odorless milk and cheese protein, used to make plastics, adhesives, paints, and foods." Plastics, adhesives, and paints? I feel like Dorothy in the forest: lions and tigers and bears? Oh my! If it's tasteless and odorless, if it's in paints, plastics, and glues, why is it in my food? I'll just have milk and cheese. Thanks anyway.

4

The Science
of the French Diet

What about wine?

If it's true that culture really does affect scientific conclusions,
you should be able to see evidence of this somewhere. Let's take
alcohol as an example. Many Americans don't want to emphasize
alcohol in our diets because it worries us – not scientifically, but
socially.

Around 100 years ago, a group of well-meaning people
managed to get it banned outright. This had nothing to do with
our health. Another group got it reinstated a few years later. That
had nothing to do with our health either. Where I grew up in the
deepest south, y'all just knew that alcohol swooped down right
out of hell, riding on a deck of playing cards to the tune of Elvis
Presley. Even today, God and some state legislatures have
banned the purchase of alcohol on Sunday. You can drive your

car to a restaurant, drink all you want, and then drive home. You just can't sell a six-pack on Sunday.

You can see this cultural knee-jerk reflex just as strongly in science. Consistent evidence over the past 25 years has indicated that wine with your meal decreases your risk of heart disease. Serge Renaud is the French research scientist who did the first work showing (back in the 1970's) what is only now being admitted in the U.S. – platelet aggregation in the blood decreases with low doses of alcohol. It does the same thing, functionally, as aspirin. American doctors are quick to recommend an aspirin pill made by Bayer or someone else, but not a glass of wine.

Doing his early work in Canada in the 1970's, Renaud recalled an American study that confirmed the exact same result. There's no magic here: low doses of alcohol keep platelets from building up along the walls of our arteries. But publication of this plain scientific result was held up because "the National Institutes of Health feared it might encourage drinking." Science had a result. The social climate said, "Well, maybe you do and maybe you don't."

Resistance to these types of conclusions, in the face of very clear data, is startling. Renaud has run into confusion from the American medical community since then. The *New England Journal of Medicine*, one of the most prestigious American medical journals, rejected publication of Renaud's more recent "Lyon Diet Heart Study." He tested the effects of a diet similar to that used on the island of Crete for the past few thousand years. They use tons of olive oil with their food, eat cheese, some goat meat, and have wine with meals – very much like the other Mediterranean diets.

The beneficial effect of this diet on markers for heart disease was striking. But the diet thumbed its nose so blatantly at our assumptions that the study made no sense at all to the reviewers at the journal. They couldn't believe the data were real. There must be something wrong with the study, they wrote, "wondering how such a large mortality reduction could have possibly been achieved." So it was rejected. A British publication picked it up and published it without a hitch.

Science speaks. Culture overrules.

In regard to alcohol, our government's official Dietary Guidelines have finally gotten off their hands and included (for the first time in the year 2000) advisement on the beneficial effects of moderate alcohol consumption. More than 20 years after Renaud's work! These guidelines are revised every 5 years to accommodate the latest thoughts in the scientific community. It took all this time for the more "prudent" American research community to publicly arrive at the same conclusion Renaud has known since the Beatles broke up.

Their advisement, though, is tepid and cautious. Wine is only recommended for a subset of women and men in their middle-aged years.

A recent story from ABC News discussed the trouble we have accepting the plain data on wine. The story pointed out that medical benefits can be blocked from the public simply because of political and social baggage. For example, an overwhelming number of population studies and in vitro experiments (60 in all) show the strong benefits of low wine intake on heart disease. You just can't get around it. An average of 1 drink for women and 2 for men raises HDL levels, protecting your heart.

In the face of these clear and relentless data, some doctors still hold out, even today. Dr. Jeffrey Alexis, from the Mount Sinai Medical Center, was quoted as saying that "because of the potential for negative effects and abuse, doctors are reluctant to recommend alcohol." Excuse me, but who's withholding Ritalin, the drug of choice for Junior High School students? Who's withholding the pharmacopoeia of diet drugs? No one.

Another study you will not hear from our national nutritionists concerns the evidence that the vitamin B6 obtained by *moderate* beer consumption prevents the buildup of another factor leading to heart disease (homocysteine). Beer also increases the blood levels of HDL, the cholesterol that prevents heart disease.

I want to emphasize an important caveat, which will help me avoid droves of irate, prudent Americans who think I'm saying alcohol is the key to health and happiness. The effect of alcohol on platelet accumulation along the walls of our narrowing arteries depends on the overall diet. It's not a cure-all you can throw at your body, then do anything you want – like people who think they can eat a candy bar as long as they chase it with a Diet Coke. You can't down a glass of wine with your Big Mac and fries.

You still have to eat good food, but you don't need to fear a glass of wine or beer as a complement to the meal. Oddly enough, like the ordinary French diet I advocate here, one study found that the tightest linkage between wine intake and decreased platelet accumulation was found in people who also had the highest intake of the saturated fat found in cheese (see the Appendix for the De Lorgeril and Tunstall-Pedoe references).

If you are French, you say, "mais oui, you 'ave cheese and wine weess your meal. We 'ave known thees for centuries, you silly Americans." If you are more Anglican you say, "Cheese? I mean ... *cheese*? Umm ... really?" But, again, science will one day confirm what we see works for the French, just like it did for the use of olive oil among Mediterranean countries. Once they do, we'll smile, nod to each other with a satisfied sort of look, and recommend that everyone do what the French do. While we're waiting on that to happen, we might as well settle back and have a glass of wine.

Also from the caveat desk, I'll add that healthy amounts of alcohol can't be put in the bank – to be withdrawn later. That is, 1 – 2 glasses of wine per day are great for you. Have a good one with your meal and love it. But if you skip your 1 – 2 glasses on Monday, you can't have 2 – 4 glasses on Tuesday or 3 – 6 on Wednesday. You'll kill your liver. Don't do it.

The problem with alcohol, of course, is that some people have a serious problem stopping at 1 – 2. If this is you, don't have a glass of wine. It's not crucial to the diet. It's only good for you. Just like most things, as soon as you have too much, it instantly becomes bad for you. Moderation is the key. If you don't think you can keep from abusing it, don't even try.

This fits with the overall message of *The Fat Fallacy*. There is nothing wrong with food. But gorge on it and it'll kill you. The same is true of alcohol, or anything for that matter. Wine is a food. Treat it that way. Take small bites of your food.

Take small drinks of your wine. Eat reasonable portions of your food. Drink only 1 – 2 glasses of wine with the meal.

The fat you eat and the fat you wear

We're gradually coming around to a healthier attitude toward wine. The same seems to be true of fat. But this change is painfully slow. That's because we're up against over 30 years of dogma supporting the low fat mentality. The American Heart Association has encouraged the "restriction of fat intake," making this the very "cornerstone of these dietary recommendations."

Dean Ornish pushes this to an ultra low fat extreme. For example, now that we know omega-3 fatty acids are good for you, he's in a bind. He cringes at all that fat you'd have if you just ate the fish. His response? "You might say, well, why not eat fish, because then you can get the fish oil directly from the fish. And you can. The problem is that the fish with the highest amounts omega-3 fatty acids – salmon and other deep water fish – are also the highest in fat and cholesterol." His answer? Take omega-3 fatty acid pills instead of eating fish. Eat pills instead of food?

But such fat free extremism is beginning to be recognized as unhealthy (see the Appendix: "Role of Fat in Weight and Health"). Drs. Vigilante and Flynn state that "low-fat diets do not work, can be medically harmful, and do not represent the best diet ... especially if they want to lose weight and keep it off." This comes from *Low Fat Lies*, another in the growing string of books debunking the old-school fat free mentality.

There are a closet full of reasons more and more doctors are coming out against low fat diets. As I mentioned before, your body thinks you're in drastic trouble and holds onto its remaining fat – it conserves it! The data for this? Animals fed low fat diets respond by producing chemicals that make more fat in the body. Independent groups in Canada, the Rockefeller University, and the University of Colorado confirmed this by looking at the amount of lipoprotein lipase (the enzyme responsible for making and storing fat) in adults on low fat diets. It skyrockets.

This is why weight yo-yos for people on low fat diets. Any fat you do eat, on a binge or otherwise, gets shuttled directly into body fat first. Even if you've lost weight to begin with, it's incredibly tough to keep it off because your body hates this diet. It works against the whole dietary theory.

On the face of it, this seems so counter-intuitive. How can it be that more fat on the plate means less fat on the hips? But think about it like hoarding. In one of the recent French strikes – a kind of routine political calisthenics – there was a shortage of gas. What happened? Everyone went to the pump and put as much gas as they could in spare containers. You never know when more will come, so you hoard.

> **You need fat in your diet so you don't have to keep it on your body.**

That's no surprise. Any gas that does show up quickly gets incorporated into someone's reserve. Afterwards, when there's plenty of gas to go around again, people only take what they need. Hoarding is as normal for people fighting a gas shortage as it is for your body fighting low fat conditions. So if you're body isn't getting enough fat, it'll grab up any new fat it does get and put it right into its storage reserves, on the hips.

It would be so easy if our simplistic notions were right – eat fat, get fat. But it just ain't so. In the *European Journal of Clinical Nutrition*, Dr. Lissner showed that the amount of calories from fat in your diet had nothing to do with your chances of being obese. It mattered not one whit, as long as it was kept between 25 and 47 percent of total calories! That's as much as 50% greater than the current dogma dictates. *Moreover, his study showed more obese women at the lower fat intake levels.* Lower fat, higher weight problems.

And a recent study by Boué and his colleagues showed that only a very small amount of dietary cheese and other dairy fats goes into storage on your belly anyway. These authors pulled out adipose tissue from the abdomens of 71 French women.

Despite the fact that 85% of their fat intake came from cheeses and dairy products, only 4.4% of these fatty acids ended up as stored fat.

Nutrition science says it's true. Population studies back it up. Lower fat in the diet does not equal lower fat on the body. Higher dairy fat in the diet does not equal higher fat on your hips. Your bottom line? Our old low fat theories are just wrong.

When fat is good for you

It's not just your weight, though. Certain fats in your diet also benefit your heart. Olive oil, oils from nuts (particularly walnuts) and, even the queen mother of dietary heresies, cheese and dairy products are important. These assist cancer-fighting agents such as the beta-carotenes found in many vegetables. These molecules only work for you if your body absorbs them, and they're only absorbed in the presence of some form of oil or fat.

Why is this? It's because these and other important molecules for your health are lipophillic, meaning that they are soluble in oils and repelled by water-based liquids. Lycopene is one of these, and plays an important role in the prevention of prostate cancer. Low fat diets make it difficult or impossible for your body to absorb them. In addition to the importance of cancer-fighting carotenes, olive oil by itself decreases the bad cholesterol (LDL) and increases the protective cholesterol (HDL).

Another in the litany of reasons not to go low fat is that all fats aren't bad. Nutrition science may wrangle over which diet to adopt, but they do agree on that. Dr. Steinberg and his colleagues, in the *New England Journal of Medicine*, showed that all fats don't end up as LDL, and even the ones that do aren't all bad. It's only one specific form of it. So eliminating all fats now seems to be more harmful than helpful.

Here's a concrete example. A recent study examined 105 men on low fat diets. As expected, they turned up with lowered LDL levels. But, as we've said, all LDL's are not created equal. One type is smaller and particularly aggressive. It gets created when your body makes an enzyme that chops up the larger, less dangerous form. Your body makes this chemical, which ultimately causes heart attacks, when you go on a low fat diet. This is how low fat diets directly contribute to the heart disease we see more and more each year.

Remember the Chinese curse, "May you live in interesting times"? Well, we certainly have seen some interesting developments. First, fat was the bad guy. Then it was cholesterol. Then LDL. Now it's one particular kind of LDL. We cut out cholesterol and later found out that we were increasing our chances of getting a stroke! We thought we could lower LDL and then we'd be safe. Chasing around after all these scientific advances gives you a headache.

Take control of your life: Use common sense

All these facts in flux confirm two basic things.

First, research that comes from an industry has an inherent conflict of interest. And beyond the rhetoric is nothing more than a sales pitch from the great and powerful Oz. "Pay no attention to that man behind the curtain!"

But more importantly, nutrition science hasn't yet sorted out all their mono and polyunsaturated molecules, and their low-density inducers from their trans-unsaturated fatties. They're making progress attacking it from many angles: basic science, epidemiology, and molecular genetics. Not only that, the National Cancer Institute is pushing for collaborations between these groups – so they can get their heads together and move forward faster. It'll just take time.

Meanwhile, I look at this situation like standing in the middle of my daughter's room, post-slumber party. A colossal mess, with giddy girl shrapnel everywhere. Somebody's got to put this room in order! I don't have to have it spit-shined; I just want to be able to see the floor.

So from my perspective, science is grounded until they clean up. We have to leave the room and let them work on it. It's their problem. I claim to understand all their statistics, biochemistry, and genetics as much as they understand why French breads and full fat cheeses lower cholesterol without making the people fat. It happens. Anyone can see that. *Why it happens* is a question for scientists, philosophers, and a slew of graduate students at this point. We could wait on them to figure it all out, but a better alternative is to turn to diets that do in fact work to control weight problems and heart disease.

Sources of antioxidants

Vitamin C: **Tomatoes, bell peppers, spinach, citrus fruits, broccoli, strawberries.**

Vitamin E: **Olive oil, nuts, leafy green vegetables, wheat germ.**

Beta-Carotene: **Broccoli, spinach, and all red, orange, and yellow fruits and vegetables.**

Source: *Arthritis Health Monitor Vol 7*, No 6, p. 13.

Americans have a long history of relying on such common sense strategies — wielding a can-do attitude for what we know works. Lots of local folk medicine, for example, worked centuries before anyone found out why. Aspirin was taken from the bark of willow trees long before we knew its molecular structure — knowing the biochemistry behind it did not make it work any better. Now it's the first choice for fever, mild to moderate pain, and inflammation due to arthritis or injury.

We can chase what science says into corn oil/margarine alleys and egg-phobia dead-ends, or just wait here for it to circle back and discover what we already knew. Moderation and good sense will save your life.

See what works. That's what we need to do.

The exception to the rule

Here's a logic puzzle. There's an exception to every rule. But wait. That's a rule too. If there's an exception to the rule that "there's an exception to every rule," doesn't that mean that there's some rules that never have exceptions? If that's true, doesn't that mean that the rule, "there's an exception to every rule" is just out and out wrong?

I happen to like this rule, so I'm going do some damage control on that goofy logic. What if we just say there's an exception to every rule, *except* the rule "there's an exception to every rule." There. Salvaged. Mental gymnastics make me tired.

The reason I brought this up in the first place is that I have a major exception to one of the most important themes I stress throughout *The Fat Fallacy*. I have argued all along that we should look to our own sense of what is right for our diet and health. You have enough natural understanding inside you to trust your gut on which foods are good for you and which are not.

The problem, as you know, is that common sense isn't a gold standard. Some of our common sense seeps into our souls from our cultural training. All the things we see on TV, hear from teachers, see at stores, and read in newspapers leave their silent footprint impressed on our hearts. These truths we just believe – our "common sense" – are personal, but also cultural.

That's the point. Our culture has made a colossal assumption for the past 30 years. It implemented a strategy based on this belief and saturated us in a thousand ways with the correctness of the idea. It was perfectly reasonable at the time. Fat is bad for you – bad for your weight, bad for your health.

Now food producers and sellers take it as the truth because buyers believe it. So what you end up seeing on the shelves is the reflection of your own biases. That's why you have only 2 choices of single serving yogurt: low fat and no fat. We, as a culture, have completely swallowed this belief.

Even Dottie – after returning from France, after seeing first-hand the benefit of a normal amount of fat in her diet, after effortlessly losing weight on the French diet, after joining my enthusiasm for this project – still had the conditioned cringe to the sour cream in our mashed potatoes (see "Meal Plans and Recipes"). She balked at the butter in the macaroni and cheese. She hesitated at the cream in the cereal. The gentlest of husbandy reminders was all it took to pull her back. "We ate more milk fat than this in France, lost loads of weight, and impressed the doctors with our healthy cholesterol numbers."

Her reaction was exactly that, a reflex that comes from our cultural training. Every media outlet has burned this sense in: from our choices in the stores to the ads touting "low fat" as the very reason you should buy their product. But this is the same kind of circular mess as the logic puzzle we started with – about every rule having an exception. The only reason the advertisers push low fat products is because you believe it in the first place. A huge reason we believe it is because we see it pitched to us in the media. Do you see the tail we're chasing?

This indoctrinated sense has got to go. We have got to break out of the cycle that spins and spins and gets us nowhere. In this case you have to see where your knee-jerk reactions come from and, on purpose, walk away from them. Ignore the visceral urges that well up from every food commercial you've ever seen. Do what's right, even when all your mother's advice to your overweight aunt Belinda pops back into your head – telling you not to eat butter, not to have an egg, not to have normal milk, salad dressing, or sour cream.

To ignore these feelings is to own up to the fact that we've been misled. Other countries, which definitely aren't fat-phobic, live out their lives healthy and thin. We've been led down a well-meaning blind alley. And it's time to get off the hamster wheel and make some progress with a healthy lifestyle that takes weight off and keeps it off.

The Reader Replies: Debra and Gordon

I am 5'4" and 145# and wearing a 10-12. I have never been overweight until the last 5 years during which I have been under great professional stress. I am 47 and Gordon is 56. We believe eating well is our best bet.

I read your manuscript and the concepts fit what I have always wanted in a diet. I also believe that social habits at mealtime create civility. So I read the manuscript and have followed it since Jan 8. What I will say about the diet at this time is that we have had more enjoyable meals in a week than in the 4 years we've been together. This really fits in with our goals of quality of time.

I'm not hungry at all when I leave the table and I find this will last about 4 ½ hours. Since we have cut out the cost for all snacks we have found it affordable to buy pre-prepared meats from the grocer (stuffed pork ribs, chicken breast cordon bleu). But what we do is buy one and split it. This saves in preparation time. We never used to carry our lunch but now people comment on how good our lunches look. Gordon left this morning with marinated mushrooms, roasted peppers, French olives, sliced baguette, and 3 types of cheese.

Having the food readily available keeps us from getting into the starvation mode. And I really can say that knowing I'm going to have a great next meal makes a huge difference. Knowing we can eat out anywhere makes a huge difference and having lost 5 pounds in 4 weeks makes a big difference.

We look forward to continuing with you and watching the progress for you and ourselves.
DEBRA AND GORDON

Faux-Foods Quiz: Picture this

There's a great story. An intrepid explorer/scientist discovered a group of natives in deepest, darkest somewhere, who had never been exposed to other "advanced" cultures. They had none of our ordinary assumptions about life. What a great chance to see how one's deepest beliefs determine what they think.

After learning enough of the language to communicate, he showed them a simple photo of himself. But they had no clue what to make of it. So he then explained what a photo was – that the "picture" of a tree, a person, or anything, could be represented on this little square of strange paper. Once they knew *how to think* and what to look for, everything was instantly visible, instantly understandable. "Oh, it's you! Right." Whereas before, it was just a bunch of colored blobs. Same data, different meaning.

Once we see the harm that comes from eating piles of chemical additives and believing the fat free hype, it becomes instantly apparent which products should be avoided, and which should be eaten. Personally, I look back and shake my head that I was ever so misinformed that I couldn't "get the picture" before.

Ingredients
Water, sugar, fructose, cocoa, caramel color, xanthan gum, salt, citric acid, potassium sorbate, artificial flavoring, sodium benzoate, acesulfame, potassium, a non-nutritive sweetener (as if #s 2 and 3 weren't enough), artificial coloring including red 40, sulfur dioxide.

Hint
This thing is almost completely fat free. It makes you feel like you're really getting away with something. But you might just want to leave it on the shelf.

5

Miracles For Sale

A wonderful woman,
Madame Usdin of Perouges, invited us to her medieval home on
one of our last nights in France. She had also invited her daughter
and their friend Natasha for dinner. Natasha had ink black hair
and Slavic deep-set eyes, and was visiting from Russia. I wanted
very much to ask her about her home and the life there, so soon
after the break up of the Soviet Union.

"It's bad," she intoned, her English in heavy syrup. "No
one knows who's in charge, you know. No one knows what to
believe." She weighed her thoughts on a scale with me at the
other end. "Our old training made our thinking so easy. You
knew what everyone was. Communist. If you weren't communist
like us, you must be bad. In your own mind, you may agree or
not, but at least you knew who was on our side and who wasn't.
Now we don't know anything. We question our enemies, we
question our friends, we question ourselves."

The ground had been seized out from under them. They had no baseline of beliefs any more. What had been forbidden was now allowed. What had been allowed was now passé. What a mess. I asked her what she thought would happen next.

She breathed in deeply, paused, and seemed almost apologetic. "A hero. He will rise up and take back control. He will make the police behave at home and give us some respect again. A hero."

My Western democratic brain doesn't compute "hero" except as a suffix for "sports" or "war." But Natasha's need for a hero was another way of hoping for a miracle. Where, after all, does one go when desperation stares you in the face and there's nothing but ridiculous possibility to hiss hope in your ear? What else is there when you've run out of choices, except to believe in your soul that something will come along and whisk away the problems, clean sweep?

Looking back at this conversation, I realize that I allowed myself a self-indulgent smile at her point of view. A miracle. Yeah right. But desperation for solutions comes in many guises. All over America, morbidly obese people feel they've run out of choices, and let themselves hope for a miracle. After all, what options do you have once you've tried and failed on Atkins, The Zone, Weight Watchers, Jenny Craig, and on and on and on? Either diet number 129 flops altogether, or the weight falls off and then bounces right back on. It's all the same in the end. The blob in the mirror is still you. Now what do you do? At some point, absurd possibility whispers its invitation to hope in your ear.

I read Natasha's hope for a hero in two lights. I know this was a last ditch psychological stab to solve the insoluble. But I also know that *this particular cure* – a sudden hero – would either be a hoax or a despot worse than the disease. The same is true of the bounty of hoax diets, served to us daily on a shiny platter swimming in snake oil. I know gullibility can be a person's last best friend. But I also know that this parade of frauds seethe around in that deep-as-a-well supply of suckers-born-every-minute, preying on the fact that these people feel they have no where else to turn.

The irrational well of hope is bottomless. And dark. So people latch onto the first thing stuck in their hands. You see this more and more. The growing numbers of obese and overweight Americans get bombarded with doctors' names, testimonials, and a fracas of competing claims. According to this daily background noise, you have a wide array of dietary miracles at your disposal.

Suck it out

Liposuction is well known. People have used this technique for over 25 years to slurp fat out through a tube. You get the image of a vacuum cleaner hose and some doctor with a plastic face shield splattered with things you don't want to know about. There's that sucking sound. Then all that gross fatty gunk on your hips, stomach, and thighs, plop plops into the sink and swirls down the drain. That's how women walk in the office huge, and walk out as the svelte beauty they know they really are.

But that's a myth on several fronts. There are no vacuum cleaners. Liposuction is a very delicate surgical procedure, and it can't take you from blimp to bombshell. The liposuction knob is not the coarse control. It's for fine-tuning your form. It's truly cosmetic, like a face-lift touch-up. That's because it can be dangerous if you take too much fat out. Only so much can be removed safely.

When I say "dangerous," I don't mean getting poked with a pipette, I mean dying from the procedure. The professional journal *Plastic and Reconstructive Surgery* recently reported that you are much more likely to die from liposuction than from most other surgeries (on average, compare 1 death in ~5,000 for liposuction to 1 death in ~200,000 for other surgeries).

You can get blood clots in your lungs, or suffer a deadly reaction to the anesthesia. *USA Today* reported on these alarming trends, but also pointed out that the liposuction procedure isn't the problem, it's the liposuction doctor. Any M.D. can throw up a shingle and decide to be a plastic surgeon. Because of this lack of regulation, the number of "cosmetic surgeons" vying for your attention is 5 times greater than the number of properly licensed board certifications for cosmetic surgeons. If you're not certified, then you're just some doctor with a vacuum pump and a pipette. As a consumer, not only do you have to be careful what you ask for, but also who you ask.

Plastic surgeons who played by the rules and took the time to get certified cringe at all the press indicating so many deaths due to liposuction. It makes them look bad. But those numbers come from the cowboy surgeons who don't take the best care of their patients because they haven't been properly trained.

Here's the problem. If the surgeon gets too happy with the suction pipette – trying to take too much off at one time – it becomes more likely you'll develop infections, blood clots, fluid on the lungs, nerve damage, or lidocaine toxicity. The maximum you are supposed to remove is about 10 pounds of fat. And that's pushing it. If you need to lose more than that, this isn't for you.

Just remember, plastic surgeons recommend this procedure for "normal-weight people." Liposuction is a means to sculpt your form, not drastically alter it.

Slice it off

If you can't just rip fat out of the body, what can you rip out? If you don't already know the answer to this, I want you to guess. Think about the most outrageously bizarre surgery imaginable. Let yourself go wild here. "Staple the mouth closed?" You're getting close. "Make a person violently ill whenever they eat?" Warmer, warmer. "Cut out their stomach and half their intestines?" Ding, ding, ding. We have a winner.

The procedure is known as radical bariatric surgery, and it is now performed up to 40,000 times per year. About 80 percent of these surgeries are performed on women.

The frustrated hopes that fertilize our grass roots economy justify this incredible procedure, which can force you to lose drastic amounts of weight. Up pops the American Society for Bariatric Surgery, a rapidly growing group of surgeons with a product, working the market. Dr. Elliot R. Goodman, at the Montefiore Medical Center in New York, was quoted in the *New*

York Times as saying "It's a moneymaking venture for them if you can do it safely and get a length of stay of four to five days." Great.

This is America, right? Good for them. But there are two other groups to consider. One is the patient, and the other is us as a society. What does this mean about us, that we have to resort to slicing apart our normal biological parts just to curb our weight? Dr. Jules Hirsch, an obesity expert at the Rockefeller University in Manhattan, believes bariatric surgery to be a radical sign of failure. We've lost. If we have to resort to cutting a person open and removing part of their digestive tract, we've run out of options. We'll know we've won our society's battle with weight as soon as this procedure disappears completely.

No one can deny that it works. Take out most of the stomach and half of the small intestine and, voilà, weight loss. Insta-cure. Tapeworm eggs would work too and keep weight off longer. It's not as sexy though. Not good party conversation either.

What happens to the patient

Bariatric surgery typically uses staples. It cuts off all but the topmost portion of the stomach. They leave enough to hold only about 2 tablespoons of food. A bypass is put in that re-routes food past what's left of your stomach, the entire first part of the small intestine, the duodenum, and part of the middle section, the jejunum.

You get nothing but clear liquids on the first postoperative day. By the third day you can have full fluids. If that's tolerated, you can move up to pureed foods on the fourth day. Finally getting back to solid food is based on the individual patient's tolerance, comfort, and progress. They don't want you to even try it, though, until about 3 or 4 weeks after surgery.

But, don't you *need* your stomach and small intestine? The answer, of course, is yes. The duodenum is the part of the intestines that digests food coming in from the stomach. This process provides your body with iron and calcium. Pancreatic enzymes are routed here to begin digesting meat and protein. Later, this digested food gets collected into the large bowel where most of the fluid is absorbed back into your body. That's what's supposed to happen.

However, people who submit to this surgery end up with vitamin deficiencies because their bodies cannot absorb nutrients anymore. This is because the absorbing part is either taken out of the digestive loop and left inside your body, or plopped into a plastic bag in a bucket at the end of the surgery table.

The effect of hacking apart your digestive system is disastrous for your body, whose entire physiology assumes it will be there. Complications abound. Dr. Deitel, of the International Federation for the Surgery of Obesity in North York, Canada, found that "the intestinal bypass operations require surveillance for protein malnutrition and other sequelae; the restriction operations require a permanent tiny gastric reservoir. Long-term follow-up is necessary."

Five percent of patients overeat and rip the staple line. Re-operation is common. The stomach pouch left after this procedure is so small that it can become obstructed unless patients chew their food very well and cut or crush large pills, including the vitamins they now have to take for the rest of their lives. Patients who disregard this mandate may vomit, placing stress on the staple line. In this situation, food may also become lodged in the small pouch and fail to be digested, which would necessitate endoscopic removal.

This cure kills the patient about 1 in a 100 times.

So roll your dice and hope you don't get a 1. But what about 2 – 100? For those who survive, the surgery works almost all the time in the short term, but not for the reason you might think. It doesn't work because most of your guts have been bypassed. That's what makes this procedure so weird. It works because of the behaviors it forces on you.

First of all, following bariatric surgery, if you eat more than just a tiny bit, you throw up. If you eat in a hurry, you throw up. If you eat sweets, you throw up. That's because eating large bites and eating too fast, puts food too quickly into the lower intestines. This gives you the "dumping syndrome" of nausea, diarrhea, and sweating. Sounds horrible.

By making you violently sick, bariatric surgery forces you to adopt new habits. You *must eat small bites* or you risk rupturing the staple line. Back to surgery. You *must eat slower* or you throw those 2 tablespoons back up. Worse, though, if you don't stick to these lifestyle changes, in time the stomach pouch stretches and stretches until you're eating just as much as you did before surgery. Then the weight comes back.

Later, I talk about the importance of changing how you eat and the practical tips on adopting the habits of healthy eating: take smaller bites and take your time. Sound familiar?

Let's review. Removing your innards works because it makes you change your habits for good. It doesn't work if patients nibble on Oreo's all day. It doesn't work if patients eat larger portions and stretch their stomach out over time. This means that the radical surgery forces people to do exactly what this diet gets you to do. In that sense, we agree.

But we disagree on just how to make that happen. I advocate sane eating habits, because even ripping out your intestines won't work unless you eat smaller portions, take you time eating good food, and thus eat less of it. *The Fat Fallacy* diet gets you there without all that blood and not one slice is made. No knives, no retching, and you get to keep your duodenum at no extra charge.

My mortality rate is zero.

Drug it off

If not the pipette, if not the knife, what about drugs? Americans looking to lose weight have a plethora of medications at their disposal. All of which imply to consumers that they don't need to take the time and effort to eat right and exercise. The pharmaceutical industry touts them as work-lite, commitment-lite solutions to spontaneously melt problems away. According to a story from ABC news, over 75 of these "miracle drugs" are either on the market already or in development. And, since 1996, diet pills and weight loss supplements have exploded in sales from $168 million to $782 million.

Here are some of the more popular miracles peddled, and what they do in your brain. Hang on. Meridia (sibutramine) alters your serotonin levels, while Phen-Pro (phentermine and Prozac) stimulates both noradrenaline and serotonin. Tenuate (diethylpropion) pumps up noradrenaline. Dexatrim/Acutrim (phenylpropanolamine) works on receptors for adrenaline. Xenical (orlistat) attacks your lipase molecules.

If you make it past the advertiser's labels and into the fine print, you find that every single one of these wonder drugs also has ugly side effects. For example, the Food and Drug Administration is considering an outright ban on the phenylpropanolamine found in the popular appetite suppressants Acutrim and Dexatrim, because of the data showing an increased chance of stroke in young women.

Again, be careful what you ask for, and buyer beware.

Behind the commercial hype, these drugs are still drugs after all. Remember the diet pills fenfluramine and dexfenfluramine, marketed as Redux and Pondimin? Six million people took those before the side effects – lethal damage to heart valves – got them pulled from the shelves. As if that wasn't enough, several hundred fen-phen users have also been diagnosed with an often-deadly lung and heart condition known as primary pulmonary hypertension.

Reuters recently reported that American Home Products, the people who produced this drug, were forced to settle their class action lawsuit for an incredible $7.5 billion. Although that sounds like some form of justice because *they* lost a lot of money, *you* can't just run out and pick yourself up a new heart valve in the plumbing department at Home Depot. Isn't there something perverse about robbing someone of their health for your profit margin, and then paying them a couple of thousand dollars a piece when you get caught?

Beyond the obvious ethical issues, as a neuroscientist, I have to raise a red flag at the simplistic assumptions that lie quietly behind this quick-fix mentality. Brain chemicals like serotonin, just to pick one, act throughout the body – all the way from your skin for pain sensation to your brain for getting to sleep. It's also linked to depression and even normal learning.

Take a pill and you bathe your whole nervous system with that chemical. Once inside, it acts on all these functions, all at once.

We simply have no idea what a global increase or decrease of this drug does to the delicate balance of your body's neurochemistry. Serotonin's neural networks are still largely unmapped. Yet we give out the drug like Pez, without a clue as to how it affects all the unknown pathways, the interactions between neurochemicals, or the bodily functions that have nothing to do with the original problem – until we try it out on patients, of course. But hopeful people take these medications daily and cope with the adverse side effects – the nausea, vomiting, rashes, strokes, and heart valve problems – after they arise.

In the end, the very assumption behind this entire approach is just wrong. If you could add one single chemical to change only one single thing in your life, like your weight, that would mean neurochemicals work in complete isolation throughout the brain and body – not as a complex interaction of hundreds of molecules in the soup. If *this* were true, then we'd be reduced to the arithmetic sum of our chemical parts, each of which could be individually twiddled to change what we want, when we want, like a biological weight dial. Do you believe this?

While we're questioning our assumptions, take one more step back and ask a very basic question. Is it really such a good idea to address weight problems with a pharmacopoeia of drugs in the first place? This treats people with weight problems as if they had a disease (like diabetes or cancer). It assumes that they are helpless to handle it on their own without medical intervention. Unfortunately, however, we got our bodies into this mess and it's going to be up to us to get ourselves out.

The circus comes to town

I grew up in small-town America. My hometown could have been anywhere, except for the local flavor given by its southern geography. We had small stores, only one high school, and we all knew a large proportion of the townspeople. If you grew up in this town (even if it was the same small town in some other state) you loved going to the fair in October.

The fair smelled like peanuts and sticky pink cotton candy. You saw all sorts of strange things there – haunted houses complete with spaghetti brains in buckets, hatchets carefully wrapped around be-ketchuped crania, and the collection of tents with weird things inside them. There were guys that probably worked at Montgomery Ward's on weekdays, but nevertheless sported two heads today, or maybe a furry wolfman face.

There's a standard routine at the weirdo tents. You get a great spiel from the animated guy in the cheesy suit outside. You say, what the hell, give him your little ticket and go inside. Your friends divide into two basic camps. One group is straightforward, laughing at how unbelievably fake it all is. The others are more subtle. They try to convince their friends that, well, he might be real after all. They talk in amazed voices about their Uncle Ed or somebody who heard these noises at his farm one night. Yeah, it was about this time last year. Howling. Full moons. Teeth and hair. I swear.

The series of "nuh uhs" and "uh huhs" always spoofed their way into laughter, all the way back to the hot dog guy. That's what was so cool about it – knowing and not knowing, all at the same time.

One look at an Internet search for "diet" and you can almost smell the candied apple stand over by the animal barn. It's a delirious carnival of weight loss gimmicks. Cheesy Man asks for your ticket so you can see your fat magically melt away in the shower, while you sleep, or while you watch re-runs. There's not a whole lot of difference between the pop-up tent carnival atmosphere in today's parade of dietary fakes and those at the fair back home. Except maybe that, deep down, you knew that the guy outside the tent also knew the wolfman wasn't real. Besides, it was only 50 cents. You could get 50 cents worth of entertainment value out of a clever phony with your friends any day.

Unfortunately, however, the fakery rooked on otherwise intelligent adults isn't playing on your sense of adventure and fun. It relies on the desperation of people with real health problems.

The Federal Trade Commission has had it up to their necks with miracles (visit their web site to see the formal complaints against these fantastic claims: www.ftc.gov/os). The FTC estimates that Americans spend approximately $6 billion every year on a fool's parade of products.

Zo-Lon and Ju-Van sound like the intergalactic enemies of Buzz Lightyear, but they actually purport to cure your obesity without diet or exercise. Slimming insoles push fat burning buttons on your feet. There's a Fat-Be-Gone ring that "taps into" the mysterious properties of acupressure to melt away your fat as if you were to run "up to six miles a day." Faja Fantastica moisture cream loses all your unwanted weight for you without dieting or exercising. There are anti-fat magnets, the svelte patch, bee pollen, a EuroTrym diet patch, the dream-away pill, the Acu-Form ear mold to lose weight permanently, various reducing belts, a sauna suit, trim-a-chin fat blockers, cushion vibrator devices, laxatives, and seaweed soaps that wash away your fat, right down the drain.

One of the keys to Cheesy Man's spiel is to make up names. Say Thermbuterol. It sounds important. The slimming soap says it comes from the "ASTER Institute of Research," which carried out a "xerographical study," and identified the active ingredient "Liporeductol Liposome." In case you can't see the grease paint or the rubber nose yet, here's a failsafe clown-detector. Look at the National Institutes of Health website for scientific research (called PubMed, www.ncbi.nlm.nih.gov/PubMed). It has a simple search engine where you can type in the name of any miracle drug you can shake a stick at, and their "scientists" too. If you don't find them, they're probably more virtual than reality.

On my search, there is no Thermbuterol. No Liporeductol Liposome either. Surprised?

Liz Langley wrote a hilarious article on all the fat frauds, and stated that people who can get gypped, should – a sort of natural selection of the rubes. But Americans are dropping like flies to the quicksand of weight-related problems. Five out of our top 6 causes of death are diet-related. These guys shouldn't be able to out-and-out lie to you about your health.

I've already mentioned that we should be wary of single shot scientific studies. But whatever your level of skepticism for legitimate science, you should multiply that times a million for the circus clowns. They say "science" in their ads, "proven" on their websites, and mention a famous doctor in some foreign country. All for one low, low price; step right in. Then they take your Visa, MasterCard, or American Express. My advice is to use the clown-detector. If the show costs more than a 50-cent ticket, just keep moving.

Where did all these clowns come from?

What a strange situation. Bozos abound, with plenty of miracles to sell. But this goofy parade of offbeat "solutions" is the very fingerprint of a crisis condition – when science searches for a new way to think. You see this most clearly in scientific history.

In addition to being a neuroscientist, I also research neuroscience history. I love seeing who thought what, why they thought it, and the real guts of the scientific process – what's under the hood – from this removed perspective.

The animal spirits theory, the first unified hypothesis of how the brain controls the body, provides us with a great example. This theory occupied the hearts and minds of neuroscientists for over 1500 years! But when electricity came along in the late 1700's, out went the spirits – scientists then believed that the brain worked through electrical impulses. There were a hundred reasons why this happened. The main one was that the animal spirits theory, as a way to think about the brain, wasn't doing so well anymore. The results just disagreed with the theory too often. Many researchers tried a sort of scientific CPR, but it was too late.

With the animal spirits theory on its deathbed, there was no agreed-upon idea around which to organize their thoughts and assumptions about the brain. As a result, more and more scientists of all stripes came up with a scatter of weird ideas for how the brain might work. The number of tried and true solutions hits rock bottom and no one can agree on what to believe.

Now flash forward back to today. We find dietary science rolling around in a similar state of crisis. And this lack of consensus within science results in the incredible florid bloom of outlandish ideas popping up at record levels outside of the scientific community. Consumers are trying anything and everything because there's no unifying leadership from nutrition science itself.

Of course, it's fine to know why we see more of these strange products now. But what's an over-weight person to do? The answer to this question requires us to relax a bit. I realize that the reason we're squinting and straining so hard to see the answer in the first place is because we have such a huge problem. But sometimes, ballistic over-exertion can be counter-productive. We would do well to take the Taoist admonition to "try softer."

Step back. Think about your diet from another point of view. You don't have to come up with some foreign Dr.'s names, gigantic words with "lipo," "reducto," or "adipo" in them, or make outrageous claims. If Americans ate the diet the French did, in the way they did, we would have their low obesity rate. That's no miracle.

Take one more lesson from history. Hippocrates, the Father of Medicine, said, "your food shall be your remedy." Don't look to solve your problems with drugs. Don't look to solve your problems with violent surgery or some stupid miracle. Look to your food.

Faux-Foods Quiz: Good try-ers

Americans are good try-ers. The evidence? I point to the success of all the bizarre products you see on grocery shelves. When the fat free mentality swept the medical community, we did just what they said. Margarine sales soared. "Food products" appeared throughout our refrigerators. We really made a good effort.

Unfortunately, we've come to find out that these faux-foods (with their hexametaphosphates, lactic acids, and locust bean gums) are more dangerous than normal foods. But the more important lesson comes in a pill of undeniable common sense. You're better off eating the real foods your body is asking for.

Ingredients

- Water, pasteurized milk, cheese culture, salt, enzymes, whey, partially hydrogenated soybean oil, modified food starch, sodium phosphate, salt, lactic acid, jalapeno peppers, xanthan gum, guar gum, annato, liquid hot peppers.
- Water, casein, corn syrup, sodium phosphate, modified food starch, salt, potassium chloride, lactic acid, natural flavors, calcium phosphate, artificial flavor, sorbic acids, carrageenan gum, locust bean gum, xanthan gum, artificial color, palmitate, riboflavin, vitamin B-12.
- Egg whites, corn oil, water, natural flavors, sodium hexametaphosphate, guar gum, xanthan gum, color.

Hint

Each of the above faux-foods was concocted at a chemist's lab bench and synthesized in a factory to replace a real food.

WHAT (SPECIFICALLY) TO DO

6

Train Your Brain

"What about genetics?"

I hear this all the time. Genes make us different from each other. If I'm fat and you're not, that certainly makes me different from you. Thus, maybe it's because my genes are making me fat. But that's like saying, I'm an architect and you're not. That's a difference between us. Genes make us different. Therefore, genes made me an architect.

But wait. This chapter is about "training your brain." It's about the miraculous dynamic flexibility of the body to adapt to our environment. So why does this have anything to do with genetics?

The wide belief that your genes determine your weight leaves us believing that there's nothing we can do about it, that there is no training your body or your brain. If you're fat, you're fat. It's out of your hands because it's your genes' fault.

I want to say that, although genetics researchers are doing fantastic work, I don't believe their results apply to every issue under the sun, including weight problems. In this chapter, I'll explain exactly why.

The genetic theory for obesity

Here's the theory: your genes play an important role in determining how much you weigh. The problem with this is that genes only change over thousands of years. But it has only been over the past 30 years or so – an eye blink for your genes – since American weight problems have really exploded onto the national health radar. We got fatter. Our genes stayed exactly the same. That's the problem. How, then, are our genes relevant to our current weight problems? And why are genetics researchers trying to fit the square genetics peg into the round obesity problem?

If you are a geneticist and you want to apply your discipline to issues such as weight, you have to develop theories that support this possibility. An important one is known as the "range theory."

This theory says that genes determine the yard in which you can play. You can go up and down and sideways in that yard, but you can't go beyond its bounds. In other words, if you're entire extended family played for the Chicago Bulls, you will probably grow up to be somewhere between 6'6" and 7'4". That's your range, which you can't go beyond. All other factors being normal, you'll never be 5'1" because you can't be something you don't have the genes for. That's fair enough.

Now apply this to weight. We hear that, because of the dice throw that paired 1 of 100 million sperm with one particular egg, you'll grow up to be a prespecified weight (plus or minus 20 pounds). Blammo. You play the cards you get dealt. It's all preset and there's nothing you can do about it because you can't get new genes. Changes in behavior will never make Michael Jordan short, or you thin, because *you can never change your genes*.

This attitude has made its way deep into our cultural beliefs. Unfortunately, it is supported by bad interpretations of good science.

Dr. Jeffrey Friedman of Rockefeller University in New York found a gene in mice that made them really fat. One gene. He showed that the gene caused fat cells to make a certain chemical. He dubbed it "leptin." One chemical. Wow. It's so easy, Dr. Friedman marveled. "Here is this simple hormone that solves the problem of how to track millions of calories over a lifetime." Solves the problem, he says.

His theory is that leptin and appetite are tightly related. Low leptin = high appetite. So, if you don't have a good fat gene to make leptin, you quickly run low on it and suddenly think you have to down 6 quarter pounders with cheese. The reverse is also true. If you're skinny, according to his theory, it's because you have tons of leptin floating around in your blood stream. That makes your brain think you're really fuller than you are, so you eat less food. It's all about the gene and the gene product, leptin. It's not about you. Your habits, lifestyle, and attitude toward your food are incidental to the genetic machinery that acts on its own, by itself.

How does the "leptin theory" do scientifically? There are several ways to test whether or not it holds water. If true, for example, overweight people should have almost no leptin in their bodies at all. Remember, less leptin, more appetite and therefore more weight gain. But when you measure leptin levels in overweight people, you find plenty of it in their blood streams.

Oops.

Even worse, giving people leptin – sneakily telling their brains that their genes are calling them skinny – results in no change whatsoever in their appetite or their weight.

Double oops.

Leptin certainly does something. Maybe it has something to do with weight. Maybe not. In either case, research on it will march forward. Especially since the giant Amgen company licensed the commercial rights for leptin to the tune of 20 million dollars. The old saying is true: when you have a hammer, everything looks like a nail. Amgen has bought a very expensive hammer, and now they really need to find a nail to whack it with.

The bottom line is that the range theory works great for things like heart disease (you're likelihood of getting heart disease can be familial). For weight problems, though, it just doesn't make sense unless you say that the "range" of preset weight you're locked into runs between 100 and 500 pounds. In that case, I'm a hearty proponent of the range theory. Those are limits you can't go beyond. But we knew that already.

It doesn't work, even in theory

Americans are almost all of immigrant stock, so nothing in our genetic makeup would predispose U.S. citizens to be any more gigantic than anybody else on the planet. Clearly the concept that a single gene or chemical controls our weight is far too simplistic. Let me give you a sense for the complication of the system.

How many times have you been told that the weather would be sunny and it turned out to be rainy? Can you name one weather forecaster who would bet his paycheck on his prediction for 5 days later? 3 days later? They will never take you up on that bet. And the reason is that the weather is just too filled with dynamic interacting variables.

It's wicked complicated – temperatures, local pressures, global fluctuations in warming cycles, etc. Plus, each factor plays off of the others in incredibly complex ways. Even with satellites – even though they can see storms coming from across the continent – you can count on not being able to count on the weather report about half the time!

Proposing that there's a "fat gene" that controls your weight is like suggesting that wind speed makes the weather come and go. Your weight results from a raucous combination of personal, social, and familial routines, mixed here and there with unknown quantities of hormonal signals, neural impulses, and emotional baggage.

The closer dietary science looks at the way the body regulates weight, the more of a riotous, out of control Mardi gras frenzy it all seems. More and more molecules are found that combine in strange and unpredictable ways. They act in a chaotic cascade to do, well, something to the hormonal and neural regulation of our weight. One day in about a thousand years they'll iron out all the scientific details.

In the meantime, since our weight problems likely stem from our eating habits and activity patterns, we should change them. The French provide a great example: no drugs, no fat free/taste free milk products, no carbohydrate-avoidance, no anorexia, no vomiting, no national weight problem. Same genes.

You can look at this from the perspective of the classic Nature versus Nurture debate. The Nature point of view says we're fat because our genes make us that way. One very well meaning older man (with about 50 pounds to lose) leaned back in his recliner to tell me that he was getting fatter as he got older because of his genes. It happens to you, so you might as well relax, enjoy the ride, and have some more Cheetoes.

> **Your role in your weight**
>
> **You *are not a victim* of your genes. You can take control of your weight without relying on drugs, radical surgery, or gene therapy.**

As you've probably picked up on by now, however, I'm more of a Nurture kind of guy. You're not a victim of your weight. You can take control of this part of your life and health. This is because your body is a miracle of dynamic interactions. And it remembers the inputs we feed into it – everything from the effects of exercise on heart rate to the effects of eating habits on appetite levels.

You are in charge. You can work the elegance of the adaptable body in your favor, or out of your favor. Realizing that you can do this is the first half of the battle. The second is simply knowing what to do to train your body and your brain.

Exercise

On one side of the universe are the people who think that your girth is predetermined by your genes. On the other side are people who believe that a person can have a range of weights – anywhere from anorexic to morbidly obese. But this second group believes those problems can be dealt with by changing your behavior.

A great series of articles in the *New York Times* on the obesity epidemic made this stark contrast between these Nature versus Nurture viewpoints. On one page was a big story about the genetic and molecular viewpoint of nutrition and their theory of the small, predefined weight window. On the very next page was the exact opposite conclusion. Dr. Eric Poehlman was quoted as saying "Our gene pool has not changed. Rather, society has changed." Fat can be reduced, and kept off, by the behaviors you choose.

The most obvious way to change your weight is through exercise. *The Fat Fallacy* diet models itself after the French customs, and so getting off the couch is an important part of this diet. However, the French – consistent with breaking every other one of our rules for getting thin – generally don't work at exercise at all. Their *bon vivant* attitude toward life would rather have you sit at an outdoor café, sip on coffee, and engage in the French national sport ... people watching. They think that if you have to work so hard pumping iron and sweating all the time, you can't be enjoying your life.

Sure, women want to be thin, but they don't want to work out. Yuck. The guys avoid getting a gut, but don't care much for muscles. Visit France and you just feel the need to relax and enjoy your life. They have a low obesity rate, even though they don't really exercise.

This is the only place where I disagree with the typical French attitudes. Exercise is important. Although the French diet doesn't *require* exercise, I believe it's a critical part of staying fit, keeping weight off, and raising your metabolism. Exercising actually increases your HDL levels compared to LDL. It increases your energy, strengthens your bones, and pumps up your metabolism. It's like putting money in the metabolic bank, to keep your body burning fuel at a steady clip even while you aren't exercising.

Everyone knows we need to exercise, but it doesn't always happen. This is because, to many people, exercise means going to the gym everyday. It means breaking up the routine of your afternoon or evenings to plod along on a treadmill. But you don't have to be a gym rat to exercise, and its positive benefit doesn't have to come from ballistic or dramatic programs.

By setting good habits for yourself, the change becomes effortless – just like this diet. Here are some helpful starters.

1) Do you know how to keep from becoming one of those old people who can't walk on their own, and shuffle around in pain just to move? Walk. This applies to everything. If you can walk, walk. If work is close, walk (or ride your bike). If the store is close, walk. If not, don't troll through the parking lot for the very closest space. Go ahead and park on the outside. It will take 6.45 extra seconds out of your day, and those steps to and from the store really do count as exercise.

When you are at work, if you only have a few floors to go to lunch or run your errand, take the stairs. You'll get where you're going just as fast as if you stood around and waited on the elevator to show up. This is an easy one.

A particularly French habit is to take a stroll around the block after dinner. Weather permitting, you can get outside the house after dinner and walk around the block with your spouse or kids. This isn't a workout. It's loving your life. Enjoy your time outside.

When you see someone who is confined to a wheelchair, or has pain with every step, remind yourself of the glorious privilege it is to simple walk from here to there. It's a luxury that is taken for granted just as deeply as it will be missed when it's gone. If you can walk, walk.

2) My wife and I have recently joined a karate class with our daughter. It's a blast. Doing some activity like that is great fun and keeps us together. Plus, it's only two nights per week. The "load" on our time is small, and it doesn't feel like exercise as much as a fun family activity. You might find that other 2-night per week activities would be fun to incorporate. There's swing dancing, bowling, acting in a play, even something like volunteering to help out at your church youth group. It just depends on what you think is fun.

The point is to get out of the house once in a while and enjoy yourself. Fly a kite. It doesn't have to be painful or sweaty.

3) Pretend you're from Mars. You can be green, or not. You can have those beetle-black teardrop eyes, or not. But think like someone who is not from this planet when you look around in your house and other people's houses. You, the brilliant Martian anthropologist on sabbatical, repeatedly see an altar in the living room. Many people have them in their bedrooms too. The sofa, chairs, and coffee table are all arranged facing this shrine out of reverence. It's elevated, often encased in a lovely cabinet. It comes with a remote.

How many times have you heard that watching too much TV is bad for you mentally and physically? You don't have to go to extremes and "kill your television" as the bumper stickers advise (although it wouldn't hurt). But just develop a healthy relationship with TV. How do you know if you are a whiney TV co-dependent? When you are run around by the sitcom schedule. When you are not free to set limits on how often you and your family watches it. If you are in control, then set limits.

Make your TV like your full fat cheese – using the principles in this diet. Pick the very best show, the one you love. Watch the show, have some popcorn, turn the lights down. Laugh and laugh or cry and cry. Have fun with the show you choose. Then stop. Turn it off. This will do a slew of things for you. First it will make you appreciate the shows you do watch by simple supply and demand (because it's 1 out 2, not 1 out of 20). This will make you value the time you do spend on it much more. But importantly, if you set this limit, it will get you off the couch. You can play a game with your kids.

Here's the rule that applies to food as well as television. Trade in high quantity for high quality.

Digression: Television and self-esteem

While I'm on my television soapbox, I have to point out a particularly insidious effect it has on your weight. Not only your weight itself, but your view of your weight. First, you generally have to sit down to watch it. So you are paralyzed the entire time – a sort of psychological opium. I laugh to see my daughter watching TV, because she's just like me. The TV becomes a Starship tractor beam for my attention. People can talk around me, but I don't really hear them. I know when to nod at them and say "Yes," "well," and "oh sure" so they'll hush and I can get back to the vital issue of seeing whether Justin, Tiffany, and Brad help the alien invaders kick their Ramen Noodle habit and save the Earth.

So the first problem is that tractor beam effect. (By the way, watching a sporting event where athletic people grunt and sweat doesn't win you diet points.) The second problem is that the people you see, the role models for you (unwittingly) and your children (explicitly) set the standards for the way we talk, the level of violence we accept, and the size and shape we want our bodies to be.

An interesting note appeared in *Focus*, a news magazine from Harvard Medical School, about the influence of TV. This article pointed out that sociologists had a rare opportunity to observe a culture before and after the introduction of American TV. The images we are so used to were seen for the first time on the island of Fiji in 1995. This report stated that, by 1998, an incredible 74 percent of girls suddenly thought themselves too fat. Many rushed to diets. Others (15% of girls, average age 17) vomited to control weight.

The effect of image is not just limited to naïve island girls. When we were in France, I spoke to neuroscience colleagues about America's tremendous weight problems. "Weight problems? What weight problems? Americans are all thin and beautiful." Of course, I had no idea what they were talking about. When I asked, they said they see Americans all the time on the television. They're all shapely and beautiful. It's amazing.

So not only do you have to be sedentary to watch TV (so it encourages inactivity and weight gain), but it also trumpets the Barbie form as an ideal, when this is not normal, natural, or healthy. It's as common as trailer parks, though, for people to sit around watching shows to see the people they want to be. But that very act of watching creates the opposite person on the other end of the screen! It's ironic and sad.

For you, in your life, you should get a sense of how much TV you watch. Then cut that in half. Your life will instantly become richer. When you treat TV as a wonderful exception to the rule, instead of a constant background level of stimulation, not only do you enjoy the shows you do watch more, but the rest of your life is enhanced as well. Just turn it off. Turn on your life. Do it on purpose. Find other things to do. This, with no other changes in activity level, will keep you out of the obesity weight range.

Digression over. Now lets get back to training your brain.

What you do matters

The popular misconception tells us that your genes determine whether you are obese or not. You are what you are: your behavior can't change your genes, so it can't make a substantial difference in your final weight. But *The Fat Fallacy* diet shows that your body dynamic can and does change its expectations, based on what you do with it. In fact, changing your behavior alone changes your weight, your health, and even your brain itself. We currently only understand a fraction of the gory details about the brain, and how it interacts with the world. But what we do know is that *changing your behavior changes your brain*, even at the level of individual neurons. Let me give you two quick examples.

Close your eyes and think about where your arm is. You just know where it is. The reason you know is because a thousand little receptors in each muscle tell your brain when you've moved – even when your arm gets moved passively. The neat thing is that they don't sense your position for you, they tell you when there was a *change in position*. If you didn't move, you wouldn't know where you were! There are patients who lose those receptors, and have limbs that "drift" when they aren't looking right at them. Our brains are set up to sense when change happens, and adjust to that change.

If you are like me, sitting in front of a computer screen for hours at a time, you stop noticing the hum of the computer fan. That's because the constant background noise never changes. If it doesn't change, it's filtered out by your brain. But if there's a sudden change in this level, you notice it right away. This is true all across the brain. Your ears expect a certain amount of noise to hear and your body expects an amount of food to eat.

The conclusion? Your brain has expectations. You can see this bubble up from the nerve cells all the way to our behaviors. But the good news is that your brain's expectations are modifiable! They can go up or down. The inherent adaptability can work for you or against you. You (not your genes) determine this. Sugar intake is the easiest area to see this happen.

Since the 1970's, Americans have increased their yearly sugar consumption by 28 pounds. That's enormous. Think about how many 5 lb bags of sugar you buy per year: 2, maybe 3. The other *(13 - 18 pounds)* comes from the sweetener additives in candies, fat free products, and non-desserts such as cereals, peanut butter, etc. Sodas have incredible amounts of sugar in them. We are inundated with sugar in our foods and drinks.

Part of the problem is that once you have a taste for 28 more pounds of sugar per year, you expect that level of sweetness. You crave that much more before your body gives you the gag reflex, telling you it has had too much sugar. But this level is changeable, too.

If you increase your sensitivity to sugar, you stop sooner. This makes it very easy to say no to sweets, snacks, and candies. You won't be turning them down because you are one of those stoic people who can turn their backs on pleasure. You say no because your sweet tooth is satisfied. You just don't want it.

The best way to decrease your sweet tooth sensitivity is to do it a little at a time. The most obvious solution is to cut out sugar in your coffee or tea. But quite honestly, this is only a very small portion of the total. The lion's share comes from soft drinks and high-fructose sweeteners in our foods.

The Reader Replies: Clint and Diana

After devouring your book followed by a glass of red wine, the thing that stuck with me was to slow down!

I have a second family of 3 teen boys, 13-19, who can put away some food. So I started serving our meals in courses, like you said, keeping the next one until everyone had what they wanted of the first one. What I saw was that everyone got satisfied sooner as the meal went on. But more importantly, it was a great time for our family to talk! This gives us a chance to enjoy each other for longer moments in our busy lives.

We're relearning to take time for ourselves with our family meal, like we always take time for everyone else. In the process, I've lost 5 lbs and feel like I have a lot more energy and do not feel cheated by my food.

Thank you for your work and your time.
Sincerely,
Clint and Di

1. First, if you can't give up regular sodas right away, don't switch to diet drinks with NutraSweet in them – aspartame has been linked to cell death in the brain (please see section: "If It Ain't Food, Don't Eat It"). Instead, try adding some soda water, or make your own bubbly cocktail with soda water and fruit juice. This gives you an opportunity to slowly pull back on the poundage of sugar you drink in a day. Your goal is to eventually wean yourself off of soft drinks altogether.

2. I love chocolate. But some chocolates are packed with sugar. Begin moving your tastes from the common sweet milk chocolate to darker chocolates that have more cocoa butter (which, by the way, is very good for you) and less sugar, palm oil, etc. Because a smaller amount of the richer, darker chocolate satisfies you, you end up eating less anyway, and you get more flavor in the process.

   If your kids like chocolate milk in the summer, or hot chocolate in the winter, that's no problem. Throw some milk in a pan and add 1 heaping tsp of cocoa and 1 tsp of sugar per serving. It's good, it's good for them, and you get to limit how much sugar they get. By the way, this takes all of 5 minutes to make.

3. Avoid faux-foods. These are always packed with high-fructose corn syrup. How else are you going to make them taste good? There is no additive dextrose in chicken, fish, pasta, tomatoes, etc. Eating real food, by itself, will readjust your tastes away from so much sugar.

Even with these 3 starters, you begin to see what happens here. The amount of sweet foods *you want to eat* drops and drops. The best thing is that getting from here to there – that is, getting your body to be sensitive to sweetened foods – is something you can work with. You are in control. You can take this as low as you are comfortable with. And you don't have to be ruled by your cravings.

Upgrade your milk

Remember that our outdated guidelines tell you that no more than 30% of your total calories should come from fat. Since 1982, when the National Research Council told us we should drop our total fat consumption from 40% to 30%, we have continually lowered our fat intake and raised our health problems. I hope I've clearly shown that this is abnormal, far too low, and downright unhealthy. You need a normal amount of fat in your diet. This will range from 35 – 50% of your total calories. Remember the studies in the *European Journal of Clinical Nutrition* showing that a range of fat intake as wide as 25 – 47% has no effect whatsoever on who gets fat and who doesn't.

This has been replicated over and over. One researcher (see reference by Willett in Appendix) stated this principle very clearly. "Obesity is primarily a function of total energy intake … the percentage of energy from fat in the diet appears to have little if any long-term effect on obesity."

But these studies were done in countries with a culture of sane eating habits to draw on. What about us Americans, stranded in the low fat world? I grew up with the fat free mentality, just like everyone else. My mom bought 2% milk and that formed my body's expectations for a normal level of milk fat. I remember trying the skim milk and thinking that it tasted horrible. Like water. I also tried normal whole milk and thought it tasted like cream.

On *The Fat Fallacy* diet, you will raise your body's baseline from our abnormally low levels of fat. To begin the process, I recommend working your way up to whole milk. If you've been drinking one of the low fat milks, you may not be able to go directly to whole milk, because your tastes have been "set" on the level you currently drink. This set point, however, like everything else in your body, is adjustable. It's not chiseled in stone. You can alter this by ratcheting up to the next level, little by little.

Say you are drinking 1% milk. Go to 2% for a week or two, until you get used to it. During this time, drink your milk, but don't glug vats of it. You will see several important things happen. First of all, you notice how good it tastes. Second, less volume of this milk fills you more. Finally, once you are comfortable with the 2% milk, it'll taste perfectly normal to you. Remember when it tasted too thick, too strong? Now if you go back to the 1%, it'll taste like milk-flavored water. When this happens, you have just begun to train your brain and body to expect different percentages of fat in your diet.

Once you have gotten used to 2%, slowly go to the whole milk. Bring yourself up to whole milk the same way you did with the 2%. You'll taste this rich liquid food, drink a little, drink a little, and then you'll notice that you're satisfied. Cold milk is so good.

Fine tune your food amounts

We have heard over and over that eating too much will kill you. There's a direct correlation between the *quantity you eat* and *the length of your life*. Anorexics aside, simply eating less food extends your life. That's as basic a fact as I can give you.

The problem with eating less food is that you're hungry. You may be the type of person who really can sit down and eat an entire pie at one sitting. That's the amount you're hungry for. But think of this amount in the same way as you think about levels of sugar in your diet – as an adaptable bar you can raise or lower slowly over time.

I have to make an important point. This diet is not about deprivation. It's not about starvation. This diet is about exchanging quantity for quality. Eating richer, better food and loving it is what this diet does. Eating fewer calories falls out naturally from that. Losing weight is the next step in the cascade. You aren't losing weight, you are developing a healthy relationship with your food. Weight loss just happens.

Now let's be practical. How do you get away from a fodder, trough-feeding kind of diet? First, follow the guidelines I set out in the section on the personal and social habits of eating. Gradually, your expectations change on several levels.

- **The first level is physical.** Your stomach is a certain size. That size is incredibly adaptable. Even people who have their stomachs stapled shut can gain all their weight back because the stomach responds to a larger and larger amount of food by actually increasing its physical size.

  But if you can stretch it, you can shrink it. And you don't have to do this by some heroic surgery. All you have to do is eat richer foods, use the habits of healthy eating, take your time, and your stomach will begin to "expect" less food.

- **The second level is chemical.** Your brain responds to chemicals because its nerve cells have little antennae called *receptors* ready to pick them up when they float past. We know that those receptors adjust themselves, depending on how many of their chemicals they get. If you have tons of those chemicals, your neurons will cut back on the receptors. Even at the level of the neuron, your brain adjusts itself and tunes its performance to what you put in.

  So put your brain in training. Make the nerve cells adjust their expectations by eating better food, slower. At the deepest, most fundamental level of your biology, you will not be driven to eat and eat and eat and eat. The neuroscience is complex, but the message is simple. You are not powerless to take charge of your biological urges.

- **The third level is psychological.** You have a mental expectation of what's too much and what's not enough. This amount can change.

  When you sit down to a meal at a restaurant, you expect a certain portion size. You never think about it, but most people have this rule: the food should fill the plate, the soup should fill the bowl. You feel cheated if you're paying good money and someone doesn't give you enough food. Some places use elephant-sized plates and, therefore, elephant-sized portions. This can also happen at home.

The solution is to put your food in a smaller dish. There's just less space there, so you don't have to serve obscene portions to fill it up. This becomes your psychological set point for a normal amount. Then when you go to a restaurant and see people choking back buckets of food, it's really kind of gross.

The message is intuitive. Develop habits that help you, not hurt you. Pull back on the sugar in your food. Ease in the healthy vegetable and milk fats into your diet. These will slowly adjust your expectations and tastes to a normal diet. You have the means within you to change your life. Take your weight and health back for your own and train your stomach, train your brain, and train your mind to eat normal amounts.

Be forewarned. This is not a quick fix. It's deeper than that. It's a way of thinking that you can apply throughout your life to achieve controlled weight and optimal health, from here to the end.

Faux-Foods Quiz: Naugahyde

Remember Naugahyde? A million years ago when I was young, they advertised this amazing new vinyl polymer that covered couches, chairs, and car seats. Naugahyde was advertised as a genuine imitation of leather. I loved that. An honest to goodness fake. It was related to cow hide, but only like a cousin twice removed.

I was struck by this very popular faux-food below, because it contains artificial margarine flavoring. If Naugahyde is leather, twice removed, then margarine is butter in some outer orbit. But now there's even a fake of the fake. *Artificial margarine*. That's some distant memory of margarine. So what, if anything, is artificial margarine *flavoring*? It's not even artificial margarine. It's an imitation of an imitation of an imitation of butter.

Ingredients
Partially hydrogenated soybean oil, water, salt, vegetable mono and di-glycerides, lecithin, sodium benzoate, natural garlic flavoring, citric acid, calcium di-sodium EDTA, beta-carotene, artificial margarine flavoring, vitamin A palmitate.

Hint
You won't find it in the store. You'll have to order out.

7

The Plan:

How You Should Eat

This isn't a normal diet book.

It does talk about weight, but differs in a couple of very important ways. The biggest difference is the philosophy that it applies toward eating, which affects not only the tip of the scales, but your health and lifestyle as well. Attitude and viewpoint matter, and this makes *The Fat Fallacy* a more holistic approach toward your health.

For example, the standard fare of diet books dissects, gram by gram, the food they want you to eat. They focus on the molecule or food type responsible for our problems. Then they try to aggressively eliminate it, block it, or isolate it. To do this you must calculate your body mass/height ratio, determine your daily caloric intake, investigate the labels to get your percent of this or that type of fat, carbohydrate, or protein. Factor that back into the maximum caloric value and determine how much of each macronutrient you can ingest. It's exhausting. And who's going to follow through on this for long anyway?

Not only is it difficult to stay on these diets, but it can't be good for you. What does "balanced diet" mean if you are avoiding all carbohydrates? Restricting an entire class of foods from your diet is a bad idea all around.

Competing popular fad diets

The difference between them comes down to which sub-component is cast as the dietary evil.

- **Atkins: carbohydrates make you fat.**
- **Ornish: fats make you fat.**
- **Steward: sugars make you fat.**

Although the bad guy is different in each case, they're all alike in one respect. They all avoid the importance of simple eating habits, and create the impression that *how you eat* doesn't matter at all. Weight control is reduced to number crunching the micro- and macronutrients.

The USDA seems to agree. In their recent report on competing fad diets, they stated that "it is the total calories consumed rather than how much fat, carbohydrate, and protein ... that is the major determinant of weight loss." Most diets that focus on a single nutrient help people drop pounds quickly, but they can't maintain that weight loss. It's depressing to read that only 5% of people who initially lose weight on these fad diets manage to keep it off.

The common sense approach I advocate is not a quick-fix remedy. You'll never hear me say, "thirty days to thinner thighs," "flatten your belly while you sleep," or "ancient herbal remedies foil the fat." I estimate that, on average, the people on *The Fat Fallacy* diet lose about 1 pound per week until they get within 5 – 10 pounds of their target. This mirrors the best-case guidelines from the International Food Information Council Foundation. According to this group, "... success depends on a varied diet, reduced calories, and regular exercise. Losing weight slowly and gradually increases the chances that the weight will stay off."

The key to providing realistic guidelines for a sustainable, long-term solution to weight and wellness is to include the style of eating just as much as substance of the food.

So first I introduce you to *how we should eat*. Then comes its natural extension – *what we should eat*. These factors, like blue and yellow, result in a totally unique product. If you want this same "shade" for yourself, you have to include both elements. Leave one out and the end result will be completely different. The whole is only available by blending the parts. If you change your eating style, but keep chasing French fries and ketchup with a Coke every day, no habits are going to help you. And if you eat a healthy diet, but eat buckets of it, you'll still get just as fat, just as quick.

While both of these are important, the habits of healthy eating are paramount. These straightforward approaches, once you hear them, will seem so intuitive and natural as to be obvious. Moreover, these sane eating habits are enough in themselves to begin the weight loss process. This occurs without starvation or overt suffering on your part, but as a natural product of your body's own regulatory mechanisms.

The details: Habits matter

Before I went to graduate school I was a research chemist in Dalton, Georgia. Several chemists and some flashy salesmen were afoot, but the most colorful of the cast were the "techs." At lunch time, daily, one of these good old boys very fondly proclaimed, "Welp, time to strap on the ole feed sack." And then, daily, he would laugh uproariously. It seemed to be just as funny each and every time he said it. I realize these guys aren't typical by any stretch, but given how quickly we usually eat our food, piled in a heap on our plates, the metaphor of the feed sack is not too far off.

The take-home message here is that we need to look closely at the habits of healthy eating – every bit as much as the molecular bits we eat. For example, I want to bring us back to the family table. What struck me about the French eating routines was that they still keep many of the same rules that Americans have long since discarded from the ever-quickening pace of our hurried lives. Holding onto their intuitive habits is why the French don't have to hyper-analyze every portion of their food.

As you will see, the approach I advocate is essentially French, but also recognizably American. I'm not proposing anything dramatic or miraculously novel, but just reminding us about something we've simply forgotten. I grew up with these rules. However, I had to go to France and back to realize how important they are to our weight and health.

Rushing leads to weight problems

The French have the most admired culture of eating in the world, with their luxurious 3-hour meals in many courses of sinfully sumptuous food. American eating habits, by contrast, orient themselves toward squeezing a bit more work out of the day.

I have to admit that I've been the biggest perpetrator of bad habits on the planet. As a neuroscience graduate student at Emory University, I took my normal mini-lunch breaks from my computer screen every day. I would walk over to the nearby fast food court to buy my burger, fries, and Coke. Then I'd walk back, eating out of the bag so that my fries and half my Whopper were gone by the time I got back to my screen. I was just happy I didn't have to waste all that time eating when I could spend it being productive at the computer. How sad. I clearly had an incidental, bothersome relationship with my food. It was something I had to do. An annoyance. This hurried relationship, of course, promotes neither health nor low weight, though it seems to be a fixture of the American lifestyle.

From a food industry perspective, the faster we eat the better. No one selling food is going to encourage you to take your time. The check arrives with the meal. The wait staff wants to know when you're finished. We hit the drive-thru so we can eat in the car on the way home. We take Biggie bites of our Biggie portions as we hurry back out the door. They even have "push-up" eggs on a stick so you can eat breakfast in the car on your way to work. That's sick.

Create this as a hard and fast rule. *Being in a hurry with your food makes you fat.* This may seem unnatural and counter-intuitive to our cultural training. "Who cares about my eating pace? It's only the molecules of food that make you fat, not the rate they're put into your body." That's why people are so convinced that pills can be the magic bullets to finally solve our weight problems. But if anything should be clear to us by now, it's that our old ways of thinking have failed. We are fat and getting fatter. It's time we started thinking differently.

First of all, old-guard approaches to nourishment leapfrog a vital issue. In any given meal, the very same nutrients will be treated completely differently by the body's dynamic mechanism if the conditions change. Specifically, rushing through a meal kicks off a cascade of effects that lead to weight problems. This set of problems is avoided by a very simple rule – take your time with your food.

This is true for many reasons. First of all, the reflex that informs your brain about how much you've eaten comes from the stomach and even the small intestine. It combines neural impulses with chemical messengers traveling through your blood stream. This means that there's a long delay between the time the fullness switch gets flipped on and says, "enough already," and the signal finally swims up to your brain telling you to stop eating. During this lag time, your body is already full but you haven't sensed it yet.

This is why so many people feel stuffed and over-stuffed after eating in a hurry. Several gracious helpings can be eaten before you realize that the body doesn't want any more. We slide well past the point of being full without even knowing it. Thus, eating in a hurry makes us overeat.

Why is this a problem? Our body naturally expects a certain amount of food, which is your appetite threshold. If you keep eating past this "enough already" point, you train your body to expect more food on the next meal. In other words, you increase your appetite threshold. Even worse, because your body is such an elegant adaptable machine, "raising the bar" can go on and on. It's not clear that there's a ceiling.

Continually raising your hunger level creates a feedback problem like putting a microphone next to a speaker. The volume coming from the speaker emits a certain level of sound. This amount goes out of the speaker, into the microphone, and is amplified; out of the speaker, into the microphone, and amplified, etc., until you hear the high squeal of too much feedback. Eating too quickly does the same thing. First, it causes you to eat more than your body wants, which makes you crave even more the next time. With each cycle of eating too much too fast, the bar gets raised another notch.

When I returned home from France, I was shocked at the oh-my-God portion sizes served to us in restaurants. How in the world could a normal person eat this much food? But, looking around at the customers, it all got consumed – with an appetizer before and a dessert afterward. You don't have to be a rocket-scientist-diet-guru to see that Americans eat incredible portions. Take two steps back and think about it from a common sense level: if we ate less we would weigh less. Again, this is a no-brainer. And it doesn't matter whether you are shoveling in carbohydrates, fats, or sugars. Shoveling is the main problem, not the food.

> **Eating too quickly makes you fat for two reasons**
>
> 1. The "full" signal is delayed.
> 2. Your appetite keeps adapting to the larger amounts you eat.

So it comes back to habits. Without them, you find yourself on the same old slippery slope of the same old wicked eating disorder: eating too fast makes you eat too much.

At this point, many people may say, "I see. My body is the problem because its feedback thingy wants more and more food." This viewpoint makes the body's natural biology a "bug" that needs to be fixed. These types of people will turn to drastic measures like drugs or starvation diets. But your body's appetite is an emergent property of the orchestrated interactions of your natural physiology, not a glitch that needs to be overcome. Plus, the very same adaptive response can work just as well in your favor.

By using the body's natural mechanisms, you can establish a cooperative relationship with your food. You are not powerless to shape your cravings, to *reset your hunger threshold lower instead of higher*. You can train your body to expect a healthy amount without feeling deprived! Best of all, training your body to stop nagging you for food doesn't result from some Jedi mind trick or drug-induced state. The most important lesson learned from French dietary manners is that good eating habits around the table can prevent the most intractable of American weight problems.

The question, of course, is how to adopt a more French attitude toward eating. We need practical advice at the table. So lets start with the easy to follow strategies of personal and social habits.

Begin with personal strategies

Eat smaller bites. Absurdly simple, this basic rule on its own will take pounds off you. It takes some retraining on our part, though, because most of us normally eat huge bites. We stuff part into our cheek pockets like squirrels in the fall so there's enough room to chew the rest without it spilling out of our mouths. Usually, "bite-size" is defined by the maximum amount we can pack onto our fork or spoon.

Part of this silly habit comes from an old way of looking at food. Our cultural unconscious tells us that, if the food is good, you should devour it like a ravenous dog. TV commercials play into this, showing people eating burgers with enormous bites and then making the "mmm"-ing sound. In others, the person is shown in fast motion, eating up everything in sight "because it's so good," and then licking his fingers at the end. Somewhere, we have begun to really believe that gulping food means you liked it.

Taking small bites, by contrast, means you are finicky or don't care for it that much. This also applies when you're invited to a friend's house. If someone prepares a dinner for you, they give you lots of food so you won't go away hungry, and you eat a lot because you want to be polite.

Once we realize how ingrained this attitude is, we can begin to change its hold over our thinking. Enjoying a meal means taking the time to eat it and make it last. That way, more time gets spent with it. The point is to eat because you love the food, not because you want to get it over with. Develop your own relationship: eating is an experience you savor and relish, not something you use and discard like a plastic wrapper. Ravenous animals gulp their food because they don't have this relationship. Civilized people take their time because there's more to the meal than inhaling whatever sits in front of you.

First, the frenzied eating habits

On a practical level, how do you break the cycle of eating large portions all the time? It's fine to point out the problem, but what are the day-to-day solutions?

- It starts with your fork. Get into this routine: **put small amounts on your fork**. Do this intentionally at first, and it soon becomes a habit that you do without even noticing. The same is true if you are eating something with your hands, like French fries, hot dogs, or hamburgers. If you are eating fries, eat one at a time. Make yourself pick up 1, not 7. If they are the gigantic "steak fries," eat a reasonable bite of one, only one at a time. Don't cram your mouth full, then reach in for 6 more. If you have something like a hotdog, eat small bites of it and make it last. You won't look like that cool guy on the commercial, but pretty soon you won't be that fat either.

- Create the following rule for yourself: **empty your mouth before you put something else in there**. That's simple enough. It eliminates stuffing and slows you down so you don't gobble your food. A number of added benefits come from this basic guideline. First of all, you chew your food better. Digestion is more complete when the food is broken down more thoroughly in your mouth. This allows your body to make better use of the food you do eat.

These rules also encourage you to taste your food. As I said before, your taste buds are only at the surface of your tongue, not in the cheek pockets or at the roof of your mouth. If your mouth is packed with half the food on your plate, you can't even taste most of it anyway. Also, piling one bite on top of another covers over the taste of the first one. This is another way that taking smaller bites enhances the taste and quality of the food you do eat, at the expense of the quantity.

- **Put your fork down between bites**. When I started looking at my own eating habits – how large my shovel was and how quickly I was shoveling – I realized that I never paused to empty my mouth before putting something else in there. More than that, even when my mouth was full, I was poised with another fork-full, at the ready, waiting on the moment I could shove more in there again. Just putting my fork down, intentionally at first, allowed me to finish one bite before ever picking something else up. This may be harder than it sounds, but don't give up. If you have a partner, work on it together and gently remind each other when you forget.

  Notice your own dietary habits – all the personal mannerisms that support eating quickly, and eating a lot. My solution is to get the fork out of your hand. Just put it down. Finish what's in your mouth, then allow yourself to pick up the fork again. It's really okay not to have food in your mouth or a fork in your hand during some part of the meal. Then you can talk to the people around you without showing them your half-chewed food mash.

- **Eat on smaller plates**. Psychology is important. Put simply, we need to have a full plate and eat everything on it. This is where plate size comes in. Food served on a gigantic plate can have a minimizing visual effect. But on a smaller plate, the same amount seems like plenty. We use the small plates at our house, which set a physical upper limit on how much we eat before going back for seconds. Sometimes, of course, we have to use the larger dinner plates if we're having "big food" (for ribs or corn on the cob or something like that), but for most of our meals the smaller plates leave all the room we need.

The issue of plate size and the amount of food you put on it reveals another hidden problem buried deep in our cultural unconscious. Many of us have a voice in our heads that tells us to eat every bite of food on our plate. There are starving children in … somewhere. Waste not, want not. Appreciate what you're given. Yaddie yaddah.

But eating to avoid guilt is no reason to eat. One solution to that parental voice on your shoulder is the suggestion above: eat on smaller plates. But what do you do when you still have food on your plate and you are basically full?

Solve the "clean-your-plate" problem

Henry Ford assured us that "history is bunk." Henry, although a whiz at manufacturing, never had a depression-era mother or grandmother who saved wilted lettuce leaves, scraped away the bad part of the food and zip-locked the rest, always had enough cans of tuna and Bisquick around to survive an aerial invasion by the enemy, or refused to toss out the last six macaroni and cheese noodles in the pan. If there isn't enough left to put in a Tupperware container and stick in the refrigerator, well, you just eat the remainders.

Hence, the clean-your-plate problem. My mother-in-law lived in a depression-era family, where no one worried about starving kids in some other part of the world. You saw plenty of hunger at home. Today, our country's opulence makes more food affordable to more people. And we typically serve enough food to ensure that everyone has plenty. We'd hate it if someone went away hungry. Just look at Thanksgiving, our wonderful national holiday representing bounty itself. Here, we demonstrate our success and good will by feeding 6 with enough food for 12.

You see the problem. Over-serving food, combined with an eat-everything-on-your-plate training, produces over-eating.

The Reader Replies: Dorothy

I must be a special case because, even though I am such a young 70+ year-old, I live in a retirement community. They cook my food for me and these chefs are just fabulous! All you can eat! That's my problem and it's made me gain some weight since I came here.

Introducing "normal" levels of fat in my diet as you describe has made it easier for me to look at that food on my plate and keep from eating it all. I always felt like I had to clean my plate. My mother told me that and I told my children that. It's nice to be free of it.

The best thing is that, after adding some cheese following lunch (like a dessert, really), I find that I don't have to eat a giant supper. I might just have a bowl of soup. That's plenty. Being so young and (soon to be) svelte, as I told you, I'm very proud to say I'm down 5 lbs in 3 weeks.
-- Dorothy

The clean-your-plate problem goes way beyond people like my mother-in-law, because it gets transmitted to sons and daughters. I hear this concern – now in its 2nd generation – coming from many of the young adults I speak with. Lisa, a day care provider in Syracuse, NY, said she could practically hear her mother telling her she had better clean her plate. She was perplexed because she ate healthy food, but too much of it. Even when the meal was over, if there was still food on the plate, she had to eat it. Nibble, nibble, pick, nibble, pick, nibble, pick –

until it was all gone. She ate because it was in front of her, and she had to clean her plate.

What's the practical solution to this problem? First of all, serve less on the plate than you think you might eat. Put food on your plate *with the intention* of going back for seconds. Again, do this on purpose at first and the habit will follow. Encourage your family to start small and then go back for more if they're still hungry. You can always store the leftovers, and you avoid feeling like you're wasting food that remains on your plate.

Also, if you've already ladled on the "seconds" and "thirds" portions to start with, it's a lot easier to just keep on eating. Otherwise, you have to get up and go to the stove and serve up another helping. Putting less food on the plate at the outset of the meal helps to follow through on your own intuitions: don't eat just to eat.

The key is to find your appetite set point. One woman asked me, "How do I know how much to put on my plate?" The answer is to put an amount on your plate that you *know* will not be quite enough, and count on going back. Now take your time eating. Listen to your body and it will tell you when it's satisfied. Often you will be surprised that, by the time you get to the end of the meal, you are not really as hungry any more as you thought you'd be. Plan on the following rule of thumb – you're eyes are always bigger than your stomach.

But what if you've finished your meal, and are still unsatisfied after eating at a leisurely pace? My advice is to do one of two things. First, serve yourself a bit more and listen in on your hunger level as you go. When you feel satisfied, not stuffed, stop. This is the quantity of food your body expects right now. It will adapt to a new level as you proceed in the diet. Don't worry about your progress, because you have plenty of time. This is a long-term solution.

The second solution (and this is the one I like), if you're not yet full after dinner, is to give yourself 5 – 10 minutes and then have a decadent dessert. Not huge, but really good. You enjoy it much more when you're still a bit hungry!

Use the same basic rules of healthy eating habits. By the time you've finished the ice cream, fudge brownie, apple pie, or whatever, you're going to be full. The reason I favor this is because if I'm full after dinner, I know I would feel over-stuffed if I went ahead and choked back a dessert. So I end up not having one at all.

Your Just Desserts in _The Fat Fallacy_ Diet.

Eat Dessert. But follow these rules.

• **Only allow yourself dessert if you are not already full from dinner. If dinner has filled you up, you don't need to eat any more anyway.**
• **Prepare for dessert during dinner by eating smaller portion sizes. This leaves more room for a sumptuous dessert at the end. A lovely benefit to planning ahead!**

Important note. Everyone knows that desserts can be dangerous. But there's a simple trick to avoid the danger. Ready? Use smaller dishes. Sound familiar? One scoop of ice cream, sitting on top of a cone looks like plenty. You eat it, enjoy it until it's gone, and you're satisfied. But put the same ball of ice cream in a cereal bowl and it'll look sad and lonely, like it couldn't possibly be enough. Typically, more gets scooped in until the amount seems right. This makes you eat more. So have your dessert in smaller dishes.

The overall amount of food your body needs will depend on you: your frame, your level of (in)activity, your internal metabolism, etc. Guys, to the frustration of every woman on the planet, can typically eat lots of food without retaining fat like women. They can also exercise it off quicker. Guys versus girls, athletes versus non-athletes, and the level of your thyroid activity are some of the multitude of factors involved. Your set point will be your own. This is about you and the amount of food your body needs to eat.

To do this right, you have to listen to your body. Have your antennas out. While you're eating those wonderful, rich, tasty foods, think about *how long* it takes you to eat and *how much* you need to eat before you are satisfied. Because your body adjusts to the amount of food you put in it, this level will drop over time. So pay attention to what your body is telling you. If you find that the quantity of food your body expects drops, you're winning already. This is what you want.

How long will this take? Your body is complex and dynamic. You have to give it time to adjust to its new set of nutritional inputs and reset its threshold of dietary expectations. I've seen people significantly reduce the vats of food they normally ate in a week's time, but others took 1 – 3 weeks before they *no longer wanted* to eat huge portions all the time. Remember, this is a sane, intuitive approach for your life, not a quick-fix "hypodermic needle" designed to artificially pull weight off. During this process, you begin to enjoy your food more as you eat less, and lose weight along the way.

> ### The family table
>
> **Much of the incessant political prattle about "family values" could be satisfied by something as simple as a family eating together every day.**

Adopting these personal strategies provides the lion's share of the solutions to weight problems. In essence, I am advising a fundamental reorientation toward diet that you have personal control over. Furthermore, these habits naturally fall out of a good relationship with your food. Don't rush it. It's worth your time.

Viewing diet as an important part of your life brings up another vital part of mealtime habits. For social animals like us, eating is a group event. As important as personal habits are, eating solo is the exception to the rule (as well it should be) and opens up a Pandora's box of issues around our dietary habits. However, the personal strategies I have covered above easily fold into the social strategies below, en route to truly healthy eating habits.

Combine personal with social habits

As we've said, the important social nature of eating has receded from our cultural view. Our world increasingly tailors its institutions to suit the individual, to facilitate freedoms that fractionate our groups into smaller and smaller units. We eat in the car, alone. We surrender the family meal to work schedules and TV re-runs. The social significance of food may not strike you as that important to your weight on the scales. But I believe it provides a vital link that not only draws people together, but also undermines the trivialization of food that leads to its misuse.

Eating at the TV and in the car

Eating in front of the TV is a prime example of how our meal has become trivialized. Staring at a screen, our food is reduced to the nondescript mash in a feed sack. We don't even want to look at it, or each other, while we ladle helpings into our mouths. Eating in the car on the way to or from some other activity is another example. While you are driving, you can't regard your food or pay attention to each other. You just reach into the sack and pull out some more fries, or peel down the paper wrapper a bit more.

Being in relationship with our food highlights the importance of breaking free from distracting, isolating activities during the meal. Think of how effective you would be with your partner if you watched TV while they were trying to make contact with you: nodding and grunting between commercials. The first step to create a healthy relationship in any arena is to give it your attention. This is an easy first step.

During your meal, notice what you're eating. Enjoy it. Think of what it is that makes it so good. What could you add to it or cook with it to make it even better? Practice paying attention to what you are eating and you begin to appreciate it more.

These are great goals when we eat at home. And this is perhaps the best place to put them into practice. But America sprawls out in every direction, and we spend a lot of time in the car. What then? When we lived in Atlanta and traveled to grandma's house (6 hours away), it was very convenient to swing by Burger King, grab a Happy Meal, and keep rolling. There's nothing wrong with this, because it only happens as an exception to the rule. Again, this diet is about a philosophy and a commitment to a relationship with your food. It's not about holding your feet to the fire over every jot and tittle of some dietary prescription. There will be exceptions, just avoid them when you can.

When you do go for a fast food meal, never get the Biggie size. As you eat your fries using the habits I've outlined above, you'll find that you don't need the mambo portion anymore. Personally, I have gone from the Biggie Whopper with cheese Combo Meal, to just getting a Whopper Junior and splitting a small fry with Dottie. If I order any more than that, it just goes to waste because I can't eat it.

Tina is a lady who had some weight to lose. After hearing about this idea from a mutual friend, she asked to talk to me. Three weeks after our first visit, I dropped in to see how she was doing. She had lost 6 pounds, but she was most excited about what it was doing for her 10-year-old son. He loved eating the rich foods she introduced, said he'd never go back to 2% milk, and didn't mind the smaller portions. Even better, he lost his incessant cravings for snacks during the day.

She related this story to me. They were traveling and had to stop on the road for a burger. Her son got his usual "meal-deal" of a big burger, fries, and a coke. He ate three-quarters of his burger and half of the fries before declaring that he was done. "You don't want any more?" she asked him. "Nah," he replied, "that was great." These habits will serve him throughout his life.

Return to the table

If the first part of the social meal is a "what you shouldn't do," the second provides "what you should do."

A wonderful friend in France invited Dottie and me to his home for a meal. Over dinner, we started talking about weight and health in France and America. So I asked him why he thought Americans have such a hard time with this problem. He said, "I think you eat so much because you are hungry." Well, no duh, Jean-Paul, I thought. But he went on. "Not in your stomachs, in your hearts."

Ouch.

Dr. Leon Kass explored this same theme – the relationship between the hunger in our stomachs and that in our hearts – in his thoughtful book, entitled *The Hungry Soul*. Dr. Kass stressed the importance between family and eating, and the link between loneliness, the need for social contact, and eating too much. We need to remember the basic fact that a healthy family reinforces healthy eating habits. But this connection is definitely a two-way street. Healthy eating habits also reinforce family bonds.

If you live with others – if you do not live alone – make eating an important part of your lives together. Remember old movies where members of a family all ate together? It's critical for us to reinforce this American

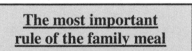

The most important rule of the family meal

Avoid eating in front of the TV or in the car.

institution. Many people less ancient than I am grew up in households where it was almost a definition of living together that you shared the evening meal. Effectively, this structures our lives to acknowledge its social importance.

In fact, many cultures and religions hold tightly to this common sentiment (the Jewish Seder and the Christian Holy Communion are obvious examples), which defines the coherence of the group by breaking bread together. With our increasingly fractured and independent lives, the time for families to come together around the meal has become an unfortunate casualty.

Recreating the family meal is important for the closeness of your family but also, strangely enough, for your weight and health. So what do you need to do to bring the family dinner to your table? The solution is to talk with your family, first of all, and agree that the mealtime is an appointment. Put it on the calendar if you have to, as an unavoidable commitment to your family. "Sorry, can't be there. I have an appointment from 6:30 – 7:30." Decide when it's going to be and then plan around it.

Before leagues and meetings and sitcom reruns, agree on a time for making your family a priority. Around the table you can stop and look at your children and your spouse and your friends and find out what happened in their day. Create this space as a consistent neutral zone where you can talk.

I fully expect this to make many people profoundly uncomfortable. Bad marital or parental relationships will collectively shudder at the thought of a space where everyone has to face everyone else. Furthermore, you are expected to talk to each other in between your small bites. Structured time together is the most important gift you can give your family, *especially* when there is some strain that needs airing out. This makes the mealtime a solution to the problem, not its cause.

The Reader Replies: Tod

My favorite aspect of the French style of eating is the time I now spend with my family in the evening. Leisurely meals give my wife and me the time to check in with each other, play with the children, and have complete conversations about whatever topic comes to mind. I have spent more quality time with my family in these last few months than I have in years.

Slowing down and taking the time to pay attention to each other while eating dinner is its own reward, never mind losing weight. (By the way, I have lost five pounds in two months.)

Thanks Will,
Tod

Once together around the table, remember that the point (as in personal relationships) is not to finish quickly and go on to something else. Of course, lists of chores always have to get done. But allocate a minimum amount of time for each other, say between 45 minutes and 1 hour. You may have to slowly increase it up to an hour, once the family learns not to gobble their food anymore. During this time, the TV is off, the radio is off, and the answering machine picks up phone calls because you are in conference – with your family! Grant this the importance it deserves.

At first, old eating habits will make the time go too fast. But like the typical French meal, rules of the table can be set that encourage conversation and discourage choking down your food. These table manners, combined with the personal habits of eating, make the meal a more enjoyable social event.

- First of all, **no one begins eating until everyone has their food**. Eating is about your family, not just you and your hunger. Waiting to begin is particularly important in larger families because, if one person sets in on eating before everyone gets their food, the first one can be largely done before the last one even starts. Then, of course, the one who's finished is fidgety to get up and go, and the opportunity to eat together is lost.
- If you have young children, you may be thinking, "Uh huh, like I'm going to get my 4-year old to wait!" But turn it into a game, and occasionally let them "catch you in the act." They will take great delight in correcting you, and as they grow up these rules will become second nature. Healthy habits last a lifetime.

When Dottie and I lived in Syracuse, we had very few family visitors. When we lived in France, far across the ocean on a different continent, lots of people stopped by for extended visits. We loved it. The rule about waiting until everyone is served became clear to us both with one particular visitor. She habitually started eating her food almost before it hit the plate, and then sat looking around while the rest of us slowly finished the meal. Eventually, we clued her in by reminding the children. "Remember kids, don't start eating until everyone has their food." Our friend now considers this an indispensable part of the meal.

After the food is served and all have their portions, everyone can start eating. In addition to the fact that this is a common courtesy, it builds patience around your food. You don't just "dive in" and "pig out." You can wait the 37 seconds it takes for someone else to have their food too. From the adult's point of view, it's no Herculean task for your children (or partner) to have the politeness to wait until everyone has their food, so you can all begin together. Treat your family as the unit it is.

- Second, **eat in stages**. If you can help it, don't bring everything out at once. Sometimes this can be difficult, like when you have tacos or some kind of food that's always served all at the same time. Otherwise, if there's a salad or anything that could come out beforehand, serve that first. Whenever possible, divide the meal into discrete courses and put them out one at a time.

I don't want to paint the practice of eating in courses as a big deal or some highfalutin event. Yes, this is a French culinary tradition. Yes, the French have a reputation for being food snobs. But the reason to do this has nothing to do with becoming more like the French, or because they are somehow more cultured or better in some way. Rather, this habit is one of the most important factors that extends the meal, slows you down, and ultimately takes the weight off.

- The third component to social table manners is to **wait for everyone to finish** with the first course before the next one comes out. This rule applies just the same if you are not eating in courses – everyone stays together until everyone is done. This is a staple of common French manners, not a habit reserved for dinner parties. Add this to the other two elements of this dietary point of view – eating in stages, and waiting until everyone is served to begin – and you accomplish the same goals for your family that you do with the personal eating habits. That is, they begin to hear their body's signal that it's full before stuffing and over-stuffing until they hurt.

Restaurants: Wham, bam, thank you ma'am!

What do you do, though, when you sit down to eat in a restaurant? With few exceptions, eating establishments commit themselves to getting customers to eat, pay, and leave as quickly as possible. The fact that you are having your meal seems incidental sometimes. Money is made when you eat, pay, and leave, so someone else can do that. You become annoying when you occupy your space for too long.

This becomes a problem for developing healthy eating habits because you'll find no quarter in our bottom-line, commerce driven economy for relaxing. Time is money. You taking extra time costs them money. We've even had waiters at very nice restaurants interrupt our conversation – *Thank you!* – after we apparently lingered too long over coffee. Time to leave.

One of the first people to try this diet is an exceptional person in Seattle named Debra, who really took the message to heart. For a special meal, she called ahead for reservations and told the manager they wanted to order their food one course at a time and spend a full 2 hours enjoying the meal. They would tip the waiter well for taking care of them, but they wanted the freedom to enjoy themselves without feeling like they needed to leave. The manager was more than accommodating and they had a splendid relaxed evening. Everybody wins.

What would it be like if this were the norm, and not the strange exception that you had to spell out to the manager? I think it would be a luxurious turn of events, that's what.

Even if you aren't ready to indulge yourself to this extent, you still need to be firm. If you can get your food in courses, ask the waiter not to bring everything at the same time. If you have a salad or an appetizer, have the main course held until you're done with the first one. This is about you, not that person's need for you to eat, pay, and leave. As the customer, you should be able to finish one thing at a time and take your time with your food.

Perhaps the biggest problem with eating out is the Paul Bunyan portion sizes. Often, you order a perfectly innocent-looking dish from the menu. It says chicken this, or fish that. But when it comes out it's served on a banquet platter. There's no way on Earth any normal human should be able to eat all that. Think of the size of your stomach compared to all that food!

One solution – if you are out with a spouse or a friend or two – is to order one plate less than the number of people there, and split them among yourselves. Decide what you would each like to sample. Dottie and I typically decide on a plate and share it between us. We may get an appetizer so we can extend our meal, but the main dish in most restaurants comes with a salad and a side or two anyway. It never seems like enough when I see it on the menu, but it's plenty once it arrives on the plate.

Another way to approach this is to get the half-sized portion. Many restaurants include this option now. This is similar to what you'll do at home – serving yourself just enough to feel like you'll have to go back for seconds. But eat one bite at a time and your body will signal its fullness in plenty time to keep you from eating too much. You end up spending less, eating less, loving your food, and losing weight in the process.

If you aren't satisfied at the end, apply the same rule you do at home. Have dessert. But don't have one if you've already eaten enough to be stuffed, or even satisfied. By ordering less than you think you need, you'll have room for dessert and maybe a coffee. And you'll enjoy them more too. This is all about giving yourself permission to love your food by exchanging high quantity for the luxury of delicious quality foods.

Faux-Foods Quiz: Great kid afternoons

Unfortunately, we have to be on our toes. Although some food products come with the disclaimer, "there is no proof that this product causes harm," this careful wording can mean many things. It may mean that the scientific jury is still out (we hear this from aspartame and cigarette companies). It states the Bill Clinton truth. There's an *absence of evidence* this product will hurt you. But an absence of evidence is not evidence of absence. The diet drug fen-phen, for example, had an "absence of evidence," before people started arriving at the hospital with heart valve problems.

A simple thing you can do to protect yourself from being plaintiff 439 in a class action suit is to substitute real food for faux-food. Broccoli has never had to undergo FDA scrutiny and strawberries don't need clever advertising to convince you they're edible – unlike the additive cocktail below.

Ingredients
Corn meal, partially hydrogenated soybean or cottonseed oil, whey, partially hydrogenated soybean oil, maltodextrin, milk, cheese culture, salt, enzymes, salt, wheat flour, whey protein concentrate, lactose, sodium phosphate, citric acid, monosodium glutamate, yellow 6 lake, natural and artificial flavors, hydrolyzed soy and corn protein, lactic acid, yellow 5, spice, butter, autolyzed yeast extract, modified food starch, red 40 lake, yellow 6, red 40.

Hint
I loved these things as a kid. Star Trek came on at 4:00 in the afternoon. I'd run into the Junior Food Store on the way home from school and grab these, cut through the woods behind my house, and zip in to see just where no man has gone before. On Saturday mornings, ultra-crunchy peanut butter ruled. But after school, life was sweet watching McCoy grump to Kirk that he's a doctor, not a carpenter; or yelling to the weekly ensign-you've-never-seen-before not to beam down, because he's sure to get disintegrated, just like the rest of them. Ah, the good life.

8

The Plan:

What You Should Eat

America works.

We have so many practical advantages of not having a long cultural history to bog us down. This has fostered our culture as the beacon of the new, the shiny, the adventurous, the brave. We are a land of laws, not men, and we act by reason, not history. What a wonderful youthful freedom this provides.

The other side of this shiny coin is that we don't have thousands of years of trial and error behind us. Cultural knowledge like this isn't written down or reasoned out. It's locked inside passed down conversations over generations. So the well-established culture, as well as the upstart, both have advantages and disadvantages.

Comparing the two reminds me of the arguments adolescents have with their parents. The youngster says pooh on the old ways. "Who cares about that old stuff? You've got to get out of the house more often. Try new things. Blow off all those stuffy habits and get with the latest new program!"

Age lifts a dubious eye. "Yes," it replies, "but you haven't even been around the block yet. What makes you so cocky? Sure, you could run off and reinvent the wheel. But even with all your wild-horses enthusiasm, you'll just end up making a thousand mistakes, then agreeing with me in the end."

It's true. Americans are young in age and young at heart. It's also true that we seem to be madly reinventing the wheel on diet and weight – and failing compared to older cultures. But we should make use of our strengths to offset our weaknesses by looking around instead of just spinning around. A bright and adaptive eye would find out what works for others and make it serve us too. Instead of banging our heads against a dietary wall, we can just look next door for traditional ways that have been around for centuries. Diets that work.

Comparing food pyramids of the world

The Harvard School of Public Health and a company called Oldways have done a wonderful thing. They have assembled many different food pyramids to compare with our own. This dietary comparison of cultures stands our nutritional recommendations beside those of other cultures. That way you can get a good look at them side by side.

First you will see our USDA food pyramid, available at the Department of Agriculture website. This is the standard information we have grown up with – the breakdown, from top to bottom, tells us the thing we should have least to most.

This is followed by three Oldways food pyramids: The Traditional Healthy Mediterranean Diet Pyramid, The Traditional Healthy Latin Pyramid, and The Traditional Healthy Vegetarian Pyramid.

USDA Food Pyramid

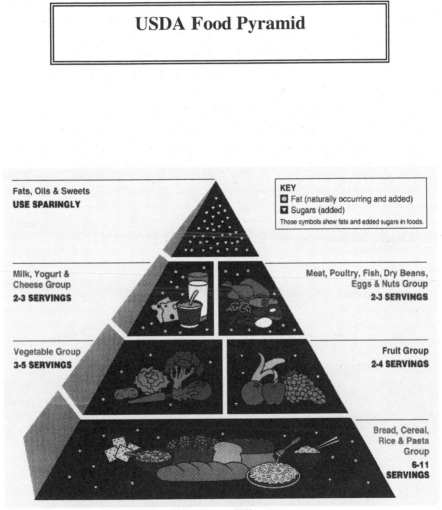

Taken from the USDA website:
www.nal.usda.gov:8001/py/pmap1.gif

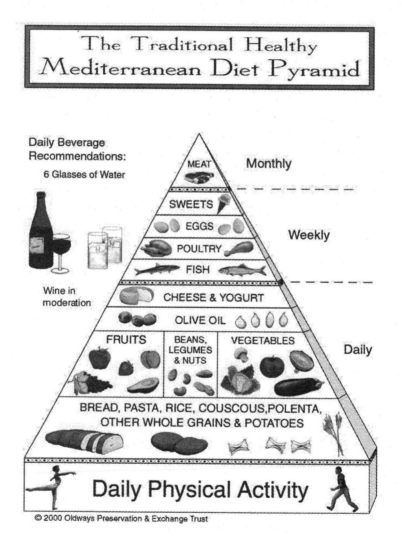

The Traditional Healthy Mediterranean Diet Pyramid

Daily Beverage Recommendations:

6 Glasses of Water

Wine in moderation

MEAT — Monthly

SWEETS

EGGS

POULTRY — Weekly

FISH

CHEESE & YOGURT

OLIVE OIL

FRUITS — BEANS, LEGUMES & NUTS — VEGETABLES — Daily

BREAD, PASTA, RICE, COUSCOUS, POLENTA, OTHER WHOLE GRAINS & POTATOES

Daily Physical Activity

© 2000 Oldways Preservation & Exchange Trust

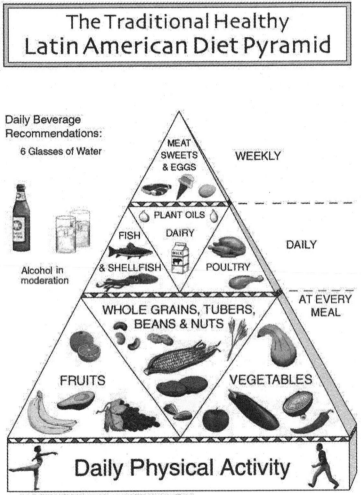

The Traditional Healthy
Latin American Diet Pyramid

Daily Beverage Recommendations:

6 Glasses of Water

Alcohol in moderation

MEAT SWEETS & EGGS

WEEKLY

PLANT OILS

FISH & SHELLFISH

DAIRY

POULTRY

DAILY

WHOLE GRAINS, TUBERS, BEANS & NUTS

AT EVERY MEAL

FRUITS

VEGETABLES

Daily Physical Activity

© 2000 Oldways Preservation & Exchange Trust

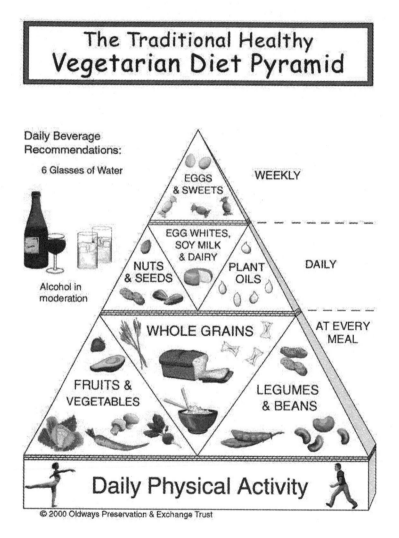

The Traditional Healthy
Vegetarian Diet Pyramid

Daily Beverage
Recommendations:

6 Glasses of Water

Alcohol in
moderation

EGGS
& SWEETS

WEEKLY

EGG WHITES,
SOY MILK
& DAIRY

NUTS
& SEEDS

PLANT
OILS

DAILY

WHOLE GRAINS

AT EVERY
MEAL

FRUITS &
VEGETABLES

LEGUMES
& BEANS

Daily Physical Activity

© 2000 Oldways Preservation & Exchange Trust

What to make of cultural comparisons

One day after lunch in France, my boss and I were chatting over our little coffees about a problem he saw with their politicians. Once they're in office, they don't seem to care much about being responsive to the voters. It seems that, in France, politicians are far less concerned than ours (if you can imagine that). After all, they only elect their president every 7 years, and the other elected officials have an equally distant relationship to the people who put them in office. Listening to him spell out the problem, I realized that our system of electing Congressmen every two years was a pretty good idea, because it really makes them have to listen to their constituents back home.

So I asked him, "Why wouldn't you just shorten the terms and make them have to face the voters more often?" The idea pinged around in his brain for a minute, considering this as a new idea, before he replied that the system's just always worked this way. "But," I said, all excited now because I had something important to add, "someone could use America as a model. They could say, see, it works for their system, it should work for us."

Oh, what a silly American. "If anyone wanted to kill a particular idea, all they would have to do is say, 'it works for Americans, it should work for us.' It would instantly be dismissed altogether." What a strange point of view, I thought. Could you really be so stuck on your own ways and afraid of someone else's that you wouldn't take a useful suggestion to your own benefit? You're only hurting yourself, you know.

But now that I'm back home and I've been speaking to people about the French diet, I find myself running into this exact same point of view. I was shocked at how many people would not consider the Mediterranean, Latin, or Asian ways of thinking about diet simply because they weren't American. Especially when our ideas have failed so dramatically, we should seek out ideas from other cultures.

This isn't selling out. It's just smart.

For example, one take-home message you get from these pyramids is the difference in red meat consumption. Notice where it's placed in each of the other food pyramids. The only thing the Mediterranean diet recommends less than sweets is red meat. The heavy political influences weighing in on our USDA food pyramids explain why we are the only ones to recommend so much meat (see section, "Political science, social science").

If you were to prioritize your meats, do it like this: eat fish most often, chicken next, and red meat least of all. In fact, only eat red meat once per week at most. The healthy Mediterranean people tell us to have it only once per month. Red meat in the diet has been shown to accumulate iron in the blood of men, leading to heart disease. This is why men who give blood regularly have a decreased risk of heart problems. Note that Dr. Atkins would have a heart attack with this pyramid. In fact, he would turn it upside-down completely.

Another huge difference you notice when comparing these pyramids comes back to our own cultural fat phobia. Our guidelines tell us to eat nonfat yogurt and drink skim milk. The USDA pyramid lumps oils together in the smallest section at the very top. They recommend just as few oils as they do sweets, and choosing "lower fat and lower sugar foods." I can go with the advice on sweets – that makes all kinds of intuitive sense. But the call for us to use oils "sparingly" needs to be reconsidered.

Why? Because countries with the highest longevity in the world (such as Spain and France) also enjoy the highest of consumption of olive oil. Fat free foods in these countries are scarce. You just can't find them. We squirm in our seats over these facts, dismissing their healthy thin lives because we can't explain them using our ideas. But the data are the data. And *these people* don't have a problem.

Note that each culture recommends we have alcohol with the meal in moderation. Everyone knows this except, it seems, us. As we've seen, the important health benefits of moderate alcohol consumption have been blocked from public view by very well-intentioned social concerns, while science takes a back seat.

In thinking about what to eat, we can be empowered by the ability to look around for ourselves. We don't have to just accept the USDA recommendations at face value. Adapting our strategies based on someone else's success has always been one of America's strongest assets. We might as well use it.

Back to our main problem: Fat and fallacy

The French eat plenty of fat, but don't get fat. Americans eat low fat, get fatter, and don't know why. A case to make the point is a young American man from upper Alabama, who visited us in France for a couple of weeks over Christmas. We took him and his family into the old Lyon district and stepped into a small restaurant along one of the narrow cobblestone side streets for lunch. Our friend, a nice enough fellow, was nevertheless a pasty pear-shaped guy who fit the caricature of a typical American locked in a perpetual struggle with his weight.

Surveying the menu, he was presented with duck liver pâté, fish something, and chicken á la créme. Faced with eating internal organ mash, an unknown, or a dish loaded with cream, he opted for none-of-the-above, and just munched on the low fat breakfast bar he whipped out of his jacket pocket. Nice resolve. But after this "healthy lunch" and a walk around the streets of old Lyon, he quickly got hungry, went into the nearest patisserie, and picked up six pastries. Maybe he should've had the cream.

Our body needs a certain amount of fat, and our cravings reflect that. Dr. Mary Flynn, a nutrition professor at Brown University, states this very clearly in *Low-Fat Lies*. "I don't believe in low fat diets. They just don't work. Fat makes food taste good, and it makes you feel full. Without a little fat you're always going to be hungry."

Given this, what are we doing? Our ballistic avoidance of fats causes people to be hungry all the time and eat the incredible volumes of food we're so (in)famous for. In fact, after only a few weeks in France, everyone in my family found themselves satisfied with a smaller amount of food on the plate. My wife, my son, my mom, and I all lost weight, despite our huge increase in milk fat consumption. We ate as much as we wanted. We just wanted less. With 50 and 60% fat cheeses and creams, you don't have to eat a lot to be satisfied. This is the key to cutting down the volume on our portion sizes and instilling healthy, sustainable weight loss. And here's the best part: those foods taste great!

So the personal and social habits of healthy eating must accompany changes in what you actually eat. We need to add in these vegetable and dairy fats. Rearranging your diet with particular foods, ironically, is often easier for most Americans than just changing our eating habits. The traditional dietary dogma has conditioned us to tweak the foods we eat: low fats on this diet, low carbohydrates on that one, low sugars on another. The approach I advocate, however, is inclusive. If you follow the personal and social habits, you don't have to worry about fats being bad for your weight, or carbs for that matter.

Eating fat free foods makes you fat

Many Americans truly believe in their Puritan hearts that you can't have something wonderful without having to "pay" for it some time. "The other shoe will drop, and the same goes for our diets." We just know that flavorful foods can't be okay.

Fat free foods, on the other hand, have a lot of stoic virtues about them. They don't really taste good so they must be good for you. Like a medicine. Because it's fat free, this also means that you can eat as much as you please. Walk into a Subway sandwich shop and the first thing you see are three gigantic words – EAT, EAT, EAT. It's low fat! They tell you that the amount doesn't matter. But does this make any sense? Do you really believe this gimmick?

Here's the problem with the logic. Our body naturally needs a certain amount of fat and craves this basic macronutrient until it's satisfied. If your foods have no fat in them, this craving never gets satisfied no matter how much lettuce or breakfast bar you eat. A fat free diet makes your body nag you for a *higher quantity* of food because it never gets what it's asking for in the first place.

Calling fat a dietary evil, public enemy #1, has caused an unexpected backlash – sugar consumption has skyrocketed. Here's why. Food companies, honing in on the low fat demand, still have to make products that taste good. If fat is out, sugar is in. Eat low fat cookies and you get sugar. Great, they're low fat! But you are also ingesting tablespoons of sugar.

Coca-Cola is a perfect example. It's a low fat drink, but it has about 12 teaspoons of sugar per 12-ounce can! Have you ever tasted a flat Coke? It's like drinking cough syrup. There's a lot of sugar hiding behind that carbonation. And on top of that, high-fructose corn syrup is put in hot dogs, hot dog buns, even spaghetti sauce. And these aren't even dessert foods!

The data are clear. Fat is not the problem. Over the past 10 – 15 years, Americans have steadily decreased their fat consumption while their weight problems have gone through the roof. The reason for this begins with our hurried habits of eating, and continues with the incredibly high sugar content in all the foods billed as low fat. Eating this stuff loads you up on more sugar, making you even fatter. You can yammer on about your dietary biochemical pathways all day, but if you eat faux-foods with high-fructose corn syrup, and then have dessert cookies loaded with sugar, and then wash them back with a coke, you'll get fat.

You gain weight on low fat foods because

- **Your body wants a certain amount of fat and will be unsatisfied until it gets it.**

- **This encourages you eat higher and higher quantities.**

- **Low fat foods substitute fat with sugar.**

To sum up, low fat diets not only make you hungry all the time, but they also throw in tons of additive sugar. The solution to this problem is to avoid faux-foods, particularly those saturated in high-fructose corn syrup, corn syrup, sucrose, dextrose, and the rest of the added sugars. Eat fruits and fruit juice if you want, because they come from real food. This is real simple.

But why doesn't the high fat French diet also make you fat? The reason is exactly because the foods are so rich. The liberal use of cream, high fat cheese, and butter provides full and satisfying tastes. This fits hand-in-glove with French dietary traditions that lengthen the meal time and serve the food in smaller portions. If the food is rich, you are satisfied with less volume. This makes the high quality of the French meal self-limiting.

I found that practically everything I had in France (except the beer) was strong and rich: the pastries, chocolates, wines, cheeses, sauces, and coffees. The French call American watery coffee "jus de chaussette" – sock-juice. In fact, it's difficult to find the low fat/no fat products so common to our stores in the typical French grocery store. They're hardly noticeable between the creams and the whole milk yogurts.

Facts and fictions about weight loss

FICTION: Gaining and losing weight is all about the amount of fat you eat, not the calories.

FACT: Calories count. If you get too many calories –whether carbohydrates, proteins, or fats – you'll gain weight. Decreasing your portion size is the first step to limiting total calories and ultimately managing your weight.

FICTION: Some foods are just fattening, like sugar, white bread, and pasta.

FACT: No single food magically makes you fatter. Remember, balance is key. You don't have to be afraid of food or skimp on quality to lower your total calories.

Adapted from "Weight Management Fact and Fiction," Jackie Newgent, RD, CDN.

The French would say, the better you eat, the less you eat; the worse you eat, the more you eat. The opposite seems to hold true for the American diet, which thrives on bags, cans, and cardboard containers filled with tons of salty, sugary things. The amount of food and the quality of food are two buckets in a well. When one goes up, the other goes down.

Now remove yourself momentarily from the normal mentality that fuels the fat free craze. Trust your instincts and common sense. First of all, cheese, milk, eggs, nuts, and butter taste great. Our bodies love this stuff. What do you make of this on an intuitive level? How could it be that a natural food could be bad for you when it's always been a dietary staple? It's like saying an apple is bad for you. If bodies crave a natural product, this by itself should clue us in that it's okay to eat.

By the way, neon puffballs, potato chips, and cracker jacks are NOT foods; you never see them anywhere in the food chain. If you want to know the difference between foods and faux-foods, ask yourself whether you can find a picture of it in a standard biology book.

What I've said so far is very general. Eat rich sumptuous foods. Go for quality in these healthy fats. Examples include whole milk, butter, sour cream, eggs – reverse the standard dietary dogma to consider these as normal foods (because they are). I'll give more concrete details in the next section, but now I want to highlight a couple of important specifics about what to add to your diet.

Foods to add

Olive oil. The ruins at Pompeii are truly a treasure. This is the world as it was – a vision heat-frozen by the Earth's sudden seizure. Volcanic sputum fixed everything in place one afternoon in 79 A.D. And now almost 2000 years later, we can be temporal voyeurs to their kitchens, businesses, and everyday trappings. Walk their cobbled stones and you suddenly recognize all the basic elements of our own life. Adolescents had a giant grassy arena built just for them to play pick-up games of whatever it was they played. Adults plied their trades throughout the sprawling grooved streets and in their stores. Even the walls still have common graffiti proclaiming a love for one, an epithet for another.

You startle at how much their lives were our lives, separated only by some technological gadgets and inventions –

such as running water and soap. And they had solutions that worked perfectly fine for them. Before the wide use of soap for bathing, for example, how did a person get clean? The Romans used olive oil. No kidding. They rubbed down their bodies, and then scraped it off with a kind of smooth metal spatula. They repeated this several times with new oil each time until the oil had pulled off the grime of the past few days and they were clean. Then they toweled off.

This gives you a sense for how common olive oil was for these people. It was used in everything, especially in their foods. They must have known, like we are rediscovering today, that this oil is incredibly healthy.

Olive oil provides a vital source of vitamin E and enhances the body's absorption of cancer fighting molecules like beta-carotene and lycopene. A Mount Sinai School of Medicine study found that heart patients who increased their vitamin E levels had 77% fewer heart attacks than those taking placebos. In addition to vitamin E, olive oil contains other important antioxidants and phytochemicals, like vanillic acid and oleuropein. These have the dual effect of increasing substances that prevent heart attacks (like nitric oxide) and decreasing the oxidation of LDL cholesterol.

Olive oil is the perfect oil and should be used as much as possible. Drs. Vigilante and Flynn recommend 8 – 12 teaspoons of olive oil per day, and Dr. Andrew Weil recommends that you make olive oil your principle dietary fat. You should cook with olive oil, have it on your salads, and dip your bread in it like Grecian olive farmers do for breakfast (see section: "Snacky Suppers," in "Meal Plans and Recipes"). And it wouldn't hurt to have a teaspoon of it each morning either.

Honestly, given the trove of health benefits in olive oil, it's hard to imagine having too much. Besides, it just makes the food taste better. Who, really, is going to eat broccoli or Brussels sprouts for long if they are not dressed in something tasty? You'll see the advantages of using oils and butters on your veggies immediately when you start bringing them in front of the kids. (For a great read on olive oil, see Erla Zwingle's September 1999 article in National Geographic.)

The Reader Replies: Lisa

I think I've lost 3 pounds already. I was Vegan (no meat, eggs or dairy) for about two years and had only recently started adding back a little seafood or cheese when I read your book. It sounded great of course. But it's taken a real shift in my thinking – from avoiding dairy at all costs to finding ways to have a nibble of cheese now and then. As you may well imagine, I get full pretty quickly with the added fat.

Today is Valentine's Day, and I've had 4 pieces of chocolate (which I never eat – I don't get sweet cravings). I started feeling guilty about backsliding or falling off the wagon. Then I realized that there really is no "off the wagon" with this diet. In fact, it's not really a diet at all. It's just a way of reintroducing food as a sensual pleasure and recognizing that pleasure doesn't mean the same thing as gluttony.

I don't know if my 3-pound weight loss is the start of anything big, but I do know that, if nothing else, I've been really enjoying my food. It's not important that I ended up making three meals out of one dinner out – it is important that I really tasted the food each time and could leave it unfinished while still feeling satisfied.

I've also realized that most of my snacking is simply habitual rather than hunger related. I've gotten used to snacking when I'm "chewing" on information for a project, or while watching television, or when I'm anxious or bored. For the last week, I've paid a lot more attention to my hunger and realized that what I usually need is just a quick distraction.

That's it for now (after a long ramble). Thanks.
Lisa

Cheese. I'm going to say it again. Eat the cheese. There, I said it. Everyone knows the French diet is healthy. Everyone knows they live longer than we do. Everyone knows this, but no one knows why. When scientists make a stab at it, they *never say anything about the cheese*. It's like an embarrassing aunt who's too weird for your new girl friend. "Oh my God! Aunt Matilda cometh! Don't make eye-contact, maybe she'll go away."

But Matilda still hasn't left the party. So you either have to blatantly look the other way or leave the room altogether. This is what we do with the fact that the French eat wonderful cheeses – and lots of them.

Brie, Compte, and Reblochon for lunch, St. Marcellin and an array of delicious goat cheeses for dinner. Maybe this doesn't make any sense to someone's complex theory of nutrition, but the data are the data. The French have healthier hearts than we do. Eat the cheese!

I'm going to relate a perfect Matilda example for you. On a recent visit to France, my wife and I were eating at the house of some very close friends. They took us across the road from their house to the goat farm. We took the kids on a petting spree through the stalls, and then bought several sand dollar sized wedges of fresh goat cheese for dinner. I was told they were for the "*chèvre chaud*" appetizers.

This ¾-inch thick wedge of cheese is wrapped in bacon, then heated up in an oven to cook the bacon a bit and soften the cheese. You eat it with a small slice of toasted baguette and a groan natural to all animals in ecstasy. I really wish there were words to describe how incredible this is. Maybe someone will invent them one day.

Until then, I can only relate what I have plainly seen. Eating decadent foods like this don't make you fat. They just don't. My friends and their children, for example, eat like this all the time and are very thin. You can look the other way and hope this fact will go away or you might just give in and accept it at face value. On the French diet, as long as you don't gorge on them, creamy cheeses will only enrich your meal and your life.

So after you've eaten, have one or two wedges of the creamiest, most incredible cheese you can find. Get the one that makes you moan out loud. Don't get the stuff that tastes like the plastic it's wrapped in or has the word "product" anywhere on it. Go to a farmer's market if you can. They're likely to have excellent choices if your grocery store is merely standard. Experiment! Have a great time. Eat it slowly and love every bite of it. They go particularly great with red wine. Road test them to find your favorites. That's the best part.

Snacks. In talking to people about their weight problems, the overwhelming #1 problem is snacks. My mother-in-law quit smoking when she heard that cigarettes addict you to a drug, compel you to spend all your money on it, and then kill you. But when she quit, she had to do something with her hands. Her answer? M&M's. She gained 40 pounds.

Here's my official *Fat Fallacy* warning label! Once you have good snacks to eat, you won't be able to go back. My daughter and I were recently in the airport mall and stopped to get a "yogurt." They only had fat free soft serve to offer. I didn't say anything, but got her a small and we went on our way. Grace ate about 2 bites and looked up at me with a just-ate-a-slug look on her face. "Daddy, this is gross!" I took a small bite. She was right. It tasted like plastic. The amazing thing is that I used to eat that stuff all the time. You never even realize how yucky it really is until you begin eating real food.

Rich foods provide twin benefits. The first, as I've said, is that they encourage you to eat slower, so your neural reflex can signal that you're full before you over-eat. The second factor is that full fat foods satisfy your body's need for fat, acting like an appetite suppressant. This works through hormonal signals that cause you to feel full longer.

This fact can be used in your favor for the dreaded in-between meal munchies, which represent a major source of weight gain for Americans. For these times, keep snacks that satisfy you with only a very small amount. For me, salty chips are horrible because I want more and more – a little doesn't satisfy me. I find that one or two rich nuts like walnuts or brazil nuts, eaten one at a time, satisfy my cravings completely. (This is especially useful if you are lactose intolerant.) Otherwise, cheeses like Brie give a tasty, healthy way to satisfy your cravings without having to eat huge quantities of food.

If you have a sweet tooth, have some fruit. Dried fruit keeps particularly well at work. If you enjoy strong flavors, Bleu cheese with walnuts and grapes are incredible together.

Now for the most important snack of all. Chocolate. The word alone makes you smile an inner smile of expectant yumminess. As good Puritans, many Americans are waiting for me to tell the rest of the story. There must some down-side. You can't just enjoy yourself without some pain in there. You can't indulge yourself and get away with it!

Okay, as much as I don't want to, I have to agree that there is a caveat – you can't eat it like my black Labrador Max engulfs his food. Use the habits we've gone over, then you don't have to feel bad about having chocolate and other wonderful foods. Remember, you are trading quantity for quality. Have a square of chocolate, not a gigantic super-sized candy bar.

Another rule applies here too. Eat rich dark chocolate. Don't eat chocolate that has tons of fillers in it, such as "milk" chocolate or white chocolate. If the ingredient list has cocoa, sugar, and other things you recognize, feel free to eat it. Otherwise, you are getting far more than you bargained for and it is only chocolate in the academic sense.

The final effect: Satisfied, not stuffed

This diet stands on two strong legs. One is "how to eat," using the habits of healthy eating, and the other is "what to eat." Putting these two together is like multiplication. If either of the parts is left off (equals zero), the product is zero. But if you include both, the result is huge, and you can finally reach the most important synthesis of this diet: satisfaction with your food. This is the endpoint, and one that you will carry through your life as long as you choose. No more falling off the wagon, ever.

Achieving satisfaction comes with several fundamental changes in your food attitude, as you begin treating your meal like the joy it is, and not like portions of chemicals that make you fat. Importantly, the deep nature of this change is why *The Fat Fallacy* diet is sustainable. To reach this goal, though, focus on the big picture – why we're eating in the first place.

Pleasure and satisfaction are the goals. By "satisfied," I mean the sense of contentment that comes from eating incredible foods, not wanting more, and not having eaten too much. Our usual eating habits, however, gallop right past this state on the way to "stuffed" – the negative sensation that comes from realizing that you've over-eaten again and have to be rolled away from the table in pain.

The search for satisfaction requires that we give up a strange, but unfortunately common way of looking at our food. Many of us think that we haven't really appreciated the meal unless we walk away packed to the gills. This mentality is why we think satisfaction also means feeling stuffed. They're always linked. But you don't have to go that far.

You don't have to be an alcoholic to enjoy a glass of wine, a workaholic to care about your job, or bloated when you finish your meal. You can stop at pleasant enjoyment by listening to your body and applying the healthy, sane eating habits to your rich wonderful foods. This lets your body find its natural weight set point, and stimulates your pleasure and fulfillment.

Hearing your body's cravings is vital to regaining control over your diet and weight. A delicate balance for many people is the tension between wanting to eat because you are hungry, and wanting to eat to have a taste in your mouth. Slowing down is the first step toward telling the difference.

But what does it mean to listen to your body? It means asking yourself whether you're still hungry, or you're just eating to eat. Are you actually hungry or just bored? Here's a simple rule: if you aren't hungry, don't eat. But to do this requires practice listening. Only then will you be able to hear when you are satisfied and avoid becoming stuffed.

As a scientist, I wince at the critical reviews that will ricochet back at me from hard-core nutrition journals. "What in the world does 'listen to your body' mean? How can you quantify something so subjective?" Most normal people, though, have an intuitive sense for listening to their bodies. We know when we're tired, when we're stressed, when we're content. These vague feelings are no less real, just because they're so subjective. We just need to refocus our attention on what hunger and fullness actually feel like. Treat it like an exercise to notice when you've had enough, and when you've gone too far. This fine-tunes our sense of satiation and helps us to see when we need to stop.

Once you can tell the difference in your own body, you have this diet for good. You have all the tools you need to carry this approach with you throughout your life. And best of all, this skill is like any other. You'll do it on purpose for a while – like learning a tennis swing – but with practice it becomes an effortless second nature.

It's that simple.

Faux-Foods Quiz: It's on your pie

Once you start noticing the ingredients of the items we typically buy, you begin to get the impression that they are all made of the same stuff. If you are scanning through these pages for the faux-food quizzes – reading one after the other – this impression really hits home. You see the very same list of strange ingredients shuffled around in most of the faux-foods we eat. Xanthan gum. Polysorbate 60. High-fructose corn syrup. Caseinate.

You get the feeling that there's one big vat somewhere, filled with partially hydrogenated mishmash. This gets put though a different Play-dough extruder depending on the "food product" being manufactured.

Ingredients

Water, corn syrup, partially hydrogenated vegetable oils, high-fructose corn syrup, sodium caseinate, natural and artificial flavors, xanthan gum, guar gum, polysorbate 60, sorbitan monosterate, beta-carotene for color.

Hint

Dottie is the pie queen. And her pies are the very reason to have Thanksgiving dinner. I think the enlightened Pilgrims sensed she might come along, so they invented this holiday, just in case. The faux-food above is often a part of Thanksgiving dessert, but I have the perfect replacement for it in the Desserts recipe for Pumpkin pie.

9

If It Ain't Food, Don't Eat It

There's a popular story.
It's about the mathematical hypothesis known as Chaos Theory. It says that everything is connected, so even seemingly unrelated effects can cascade their way from pebble to avalanche with alarming force and speed. The flap of a butterfly's wings in Rio de Janeiro, the story goes, can contribute to hurricanes in Florida. That's math for you, but the larger point is well taken. Something that happens in one place can have long lasting effects far down the road.

This is just as true for people. A man I knew and admired very much, named Jack, served in WWII and carried an unfortunate hatred for the Japanese until the day he died. He kept this feeling mostly to himself, unless you mentioned something about the success of Japanese cars or technology. Then you'd hear it. He couldn't believe you'd invest in a country that "snuck up on our boys when they's at church. Sunday morning!" He never bought anything from Toyota, Fuji, or Sony because of his tenacious emotions. He had his mind made up and he had a long memory, to the day he died.

Even if we don't have any deep-seated xenophobias lurking around in our darkest closets, we all have this same tenacity to know something just because we know it – no matter what anyone says. It's a belief, really, immune to reason. When I was a kid, my mom told me never to put hot water in a pot to boil. You start from cold water. "Why mom? What's the difference?" She looked at me like I'd just asked her why we get up in the morning and go to sleep at night. "You just do. That's all," she said, exasperated. Even now, even though I don't know why, even though it seems daft, I fill a pan with cold water if I'm going to boil it.

This "just because it's true and I don't know why" attitude pops up over and over when I talk about adding rich foods back into our fat-deprived diets. I instantly become the Creature from the Black Lagoon to people who have been taught to stay inside the little box they grew up in. The box is called "fat free," and gets confirmed by a thousand store products and TV ads. I've already talked in detail about the need to think outside this box, but there's another effect of this blind belief.

Let's say you're like Jack and you just know something is gospel and no one's going to tell you differently. You believe down to your house slippers that any fat you eat will pack on the pounds, right before it drops you dead on the kitchen linoleum from clogged arteries that doctors will have to clean out with a Roto-Rooter. If this is you, then you've spent a large chunk of time scrambling around looking for solutions inside that box. You, and millions of Americans like you, shop for foods, snacks, drinks, and condiments that have little or no fat in them.

In 1995, a survey by the Food Marketing Institute showed that ¾ of all shoppers filled their baskets based on how much fat their foods contained. Another survey by the Calorie Control Council showed that 90% of U.S. adults consumed low fat foods.

Our food manufacturers smell this demand like sharks smell blood. So fat free items show up on every shelf. This reinforces the sense that eating fat free must be the right thing to do. Our belief then confirms the marketing sense of the producers. Now we have a tidy circle. The result is a supply of foods to choose from that food companies think we demand. This self-fulfilling prophesy makes it very hard to see our own logical misstep.

Let me be clear. Our market economy isn't the problem. The problem is that we've created a fictitious paper monster named "fat is bad for you." And now we cower and cringe because we believe it's real. This does two very bad things.

1. It steers us away from healthy foods like nuts, olive oil, cheese, and milk.
2. In our fear, we do whatever our ferocious origami creation tells us. In this case, it says we need to buy faux-foods and eat them because this will save us from eating fat in our diet. It's like a ventriloquist taking his own puppet's sage advice.

But this authoritative voice telling you to eat fat free is your own. It comes from the culture we have helped create. Don't believe that dummy on your hand, because he's going to tell you to eat faux-foods and diet drugs. He's going to tell you that synthesized products are better than normal food. Remember, the fat free emperor not only has no clothes, but he's fat too. I want to raise the hood off some of the incredible food products we're told to eat.

What you should avoid

In the preceding chapters, I set out things you should eat. Now I want to mention what you should avoid. Once again, I'm not going to make an exhaustive list for you to blindly follow. I give you plenty of room inside some general guidelines to find the balance your body wants.

The first rule: if it's natural, it's okay. That's not too hard. If it's processed, don't eat it.

A Field Guide to the Best Foods, Great Foods, and Faux-Foods

Best Foods:
Anything without a label. Bread. An apple. Chicken. Like that.

Great Foods:
Things that you recognize, even with a label on it. Milk. Cheese. Olive oil. Pasta. Butter. You know what I'm saying. Nothing processed. Anything that comes from nature. Low fat milk does not come from low fat cows.

Faux-Foods:
Butterfinger balls are not food. Miracle Whip is not food. Cheez-its are not food. Partially hydrogenated oil is processed – not a food. High-fructose corn syrup? Please!

Eat food!

This can't be helped all the time. Who doesn't like a good hot dog? But what, if anything, is a hot dog anyway? It's some kind of meat mash with enough nitrates to survive a nuclear winter. In cases like this, limit how much you give to yourself and your children. Have them as an exception or treat. Don't buy something if you can't say what it is.

How do you know which foods to avoid? Think about walking around outside in nature. If you picked something up and looked at it, puzzled because you had no clue as to what it was, would you eat it? Of course not. I've told both Grace and Ben this since they were old enough to understand. If you can't identify it as definitely food, then certainly don't put it in your mouth. If your cheese wrapper says "product" somewhere on it, don't eat it. If it's been chemically altered to remove part of its natural milk fat, don't eat it. Cheetoes, for example, used to be personal favorite of mine, but I have no idea what's in them. What is "red-40"? It's a dye. Right. But what is that?

The same goes for drinks. If you don't know what it is, don't drink it. Just try to say the ingredients on the back of a can of bubbly black, clear, or neon cola. Read the labels and you often see lactic acid in there – that's the muscle toxin that gives you cramps when you exercise. Another one is phosphoric acid. As a research chemist, I had to keep this stuff under the hood if I was even going to take the lid off.

Thirsty? Have fruit juice, tea, or water. Need something to go with your meal? Any one of the above will do, plus milk, coffee, or wine. You know what these are, and you don't have to worry that someone's laced them with lactic acid.

This rule applies to other prepackaged "foods." Cut all these things out of your diet, as much as you can. This includes things like potted meat, aerosol cheese food, and fake eggs. Foods out of cans are not bad if any ordinary 6-year-old could look at it and tell you what it is. "Beans, mommy. And those are peaches." Ask a 6-year-old what Spam is (or a 46-year-old for that matter).

Olestra

If you still believe the fat free mantra, and you're in a weekly frenzy to find some way to get good taste without any fat, Olestra is your answer. It's a magic bullet. You can eat all you want and it'll never make you fat. All the goodness, none of the consequences. After all (careful, sarcasm curves ahead) the manufacturers say it's safe, so it must be. They wouldn't sell a product without disclosing harmful or embarrassing side effects, because that just wouldn't be fair.

The FDA approved Olestra on January 24, 1998. This chemical is a sucrose polyester (just when you thought polyester was out for good). That is, it's an amalgam of cottonseed and soybean oils surrounding a core of sugar. Here's the problem (it's a benefit if you're spinning this product for Procter and Gamble).

Your body won't touch this chemical – it isn't taken up by the digestive system. In one side, out the other.

That wouldn't be so bad if that were the end of the story. But this "miracle fat" doesn't just flush through your body. It carries your nutrients with it. Even though Procter and Gamble, feet to the fire, admit this is true, they write it off as unimportant! They say it makes no difference that you're losing fat-soluble vitamins and beta-carotenes. They say this despite overwhelming evidence that the carotenes in vegetables fight cancer, and decrease the chance of macular degeneration in the elderly.

The company making the chemical keeps telling us it's safe. On the other side, though, we find the Center for Science in the Public Interest and the Harvard School of Public Health. They aren't so rosy about Olestra. The reason is precisely because Olestra acts like a sponge for carotenoids and lycopene. That's why the manufacturer has been required to warn that you must supplement your diet with vitamins. Why? Because eating Olestra induces a vitamin deficiency on only a few Olestra potato chips per day (16 of them). Remember, it's not food if they are forced to paste a warning label on it.

If you are still too young and invincible to worry about cancer or vitamin deficiencies, consider this. You are at a party, downing Olestra chips and getting to know the person beside you when a sudden urge comes up (or down, in this case). Olestra can cause "fecal urgency." Great. Back to the toilet.

When you return, again, you join up with your friend who wonders why you've been spending so much time in the bathroom. But it gets worse. You can also, sitting on that bar stool getting ready to make your best move, get a greasy "anal leakage" of liquid Olestra right through to your shorts. And have a nice day.

All this comes from the misguided attempt to banish fat from your diet at all costs. Sorry, this makes no sense.

From the Center for Science in the Public Interest

Food additives to avoid:

- <u>Acesulfame K</u>, also known as Sunette or Sweet One. It's been shown to cause cancer in lab animals.
- <u>Artificial colorings and dyes</u>: The people who make them call them "inert." They have long been suspected of causing a host of biological problems (see <u>Dyes</u> below).
- <u>Aspartame</u> passed FDA muster on the 3rd try, despite repeated evidence of neuronal damage in the developing nervous system.
- <u>BHA & BHT</u> are preservatives put in foods to keep them on the shelf forever. California recently listed them as carcinogens.
- <u>Nitrite and Nitrate</u> are preservatives. In the recipe book, "how to whip up a whopping good cancer," you'll find instructions to fry processed meats at very high temperatures. This converts nitrites to nitrosamines. Nitrosamines are cancer generators.
- <u>Olestra</u> miracle fat, according to the Harvard School of Public Health, likely contributes to "several thousand unnecessary deaths each year from lung and prostate cancers, heart disease, and hundreds of additional cases of blindness in the elderly due to macular degeneration."
- <u>Potassium Bromate</u>, used in breads, is banned in every country in the world except the U.S. and Japan.
- <u>Saccharin</u> has warned you since the 1970's that it'll give you cancer. Don't do it.
- <u>Sulfites</u> are more chemicals sprinkled in to keep things on the shelf forever, and can be very allergenic. They are also put into wine and can give you a wicked headache.

Dyes in the food

So what's wrong with a little red #40, blue #1, and yellow #6 anyway? If you read what the manufacturers say, these ingredients are supposed to be "inert." Dyes are put in almost everything we feed our kids. Colors-followed-by-numbers are laced through all their medicines. Anything neon or marketed to children will have a healthy dose of them. Note: please don't believe what manufacturers say about the safety of their product – their reason for existence is to sell it to you. If you hear 3 or 4 independent sources say it's safe, that's a different matter.

Here's what you won't hear from them. Yellow #5 and #6 cause anaphylactoid reactions, angioedema, and contact dermatitis. They cross react with aspirin, acetaminophen, and sodium benzoate. Blue #1 and #2 are triphenylmethane dyes. Do you want to eat that? It causes bronchoconstriction in asthmatic patients.

In a recent article, Dr. Caucino and her colleagues reported on a specific case, in which a lady had severe allergic reactions to the cocktail of dyes (red #40 added to D&C #27) that a pill maker put in one of her prescribed medications. After extensive testing, the doctors determined that the new mixture of dyes, not the medication, had caused her problems. Reactions such as this are common, especially to yellow #5 (tartrazine), yellow #6 (sunset yellow), red #5 (amaranth), blue #6 (brilliant blue), red #3 (erythrosine), and blue #2 (indigotin).

I realize that medicines are different. I'll give my daughter the cherry stuff if she has a fever and that's all I can find. This is something we can't skimp on. What we can do is try to find medicines without the dyes.

Remember, we did not develop as animals eating from D&C yellow #6 bushes. No apple ever dropped from the branch with red #40 in it, or amaranth, or tartrazine for that matter. If you eat food, you'll never have this problem because no chicken is chock-full of blue #5 (unless, of course, he's spent time in the genetic engineering lab).

High-fructose corn syrup

In the American dietary play, fat got cast in the leading role as the bad guy. As a result, sugars haven't gotten a ton of attention. If the label says "fat free," many people think you can eat a dump truck full of it – and advertisements tell you this – without any adverse reactions to your weight or health. In the shadow of our cultural intoxication with fat free diets, the use of high-fructose corn syrup has gone through the roof, increasing an incredible 700% over the past 20 years! It's not surprising, then, that Americans have gotten fatter by the year.

It's sad to see people practically bathing in sugar and scratching their heads as to why their weight has spiraled so far out of their control. Sugar is a major component of practically every processed food you can buy. Why do they put it in there? Of course it's to attract you. Plus, it's fat free! But, then again, Coke is fat free too.

This is where weight gain happens for most Americans. As we discussed in the previous chapter, if you limit your sugars to foods, avoiding faux-foods, you will find that your taste for sugar will change. Your body's inherent flexibility alters how much it wants during the day. This causes your sugar gag reflex level to become much more sensitive. This will serve you well when you suddenly try a cola with your Wendy's meal-deal and think, "Yuck, that's sweet." When you reach this point, you'll have taken a major step toward increasing the length and quality of your life.

But it's a problem not just because it happens to make you fat, or that your newfound girth causes newfound health problems. The high fructose levels elevate your triglycerides, your total cholesterol, uric acid, and even your LDL counts. Not just in the short term, either. Yet another recent study has shown elevated serum triglycerides as a result of diets high in fructose (see "High-fructose corn syrup" references in Appendix). Triglycerides represent a key ingredient in any good recipe for cancer.

A recent study by Drs. Milne and Nielsen showed that our bodies respond to high-fructose corn syrup by changing the balance of minerals you keep and those you excrete. That is, you alter your normal regulation of magnesium, calcium, and phosphorus. This is why experimental animals fed high-fructose corn syrup develop kidney calcifications. And it's also why the Milne and Nielsen study showed that men with an already low magnesium balance are depleted even more when they include high-fructose corn syrup in their diet.

The sour things sweeteners can do

Here is a growing list of problems with artificial sweeteners reported in the scientific literature:

- **Aspartame** – Angioedema, urticaria, and renal tubular acidosis (and it gets worse: see below).
- **Glycerin** – Irritant to gastrointestinal mucosa, and problems for the metabolism, and the central nervous system.
- **Lactose** – Diarrhea, malabsorption, vomiting, flatulence, jaundice, and cataracts.
- **Mannitol** – Anaphylactoid reactions.
- **Sorbitol** – Large amounts can cause abdominal pain, flatulence, and osmotic diarrhea.
- **Xylitol** – Osmotic diarrhea.

Adapted from Table 6, Kumar et al., *Clinical Pediatrics*.

Their conclusion: "The lower retention of calcium and greater losses of phosphorus when large amounts of fructose were fed ... suggests an adverse impact on bone health if the trend continued over a longer period. ... This trend seems to be the most dramatic in children in the U.S., who are consuming large amounts of soft drinks containing high-fructose corn syrup."

Women should do whatever they can to guard the integrity of their bones. Depleting stores of calcium isn't one of them.

Aspartame: A sweet toxin

Olestra is put in the food to make it fat free. Dyes are added to make it appear as though it were something you might eat. Other drugs are sprinkled in to make the food tasty. Aspartame, for example, is the most popular sweetener on the planet. We see it most frequently packaged in sugar free drinks and in those little sky blue packets. As you can imagine from the economic investment poured into this chemical, the issue over whether or not it's healthy will be hotly debated.

So what's wrong with aspartame? Once inside your body, it breaks down to aspartate, an excitatory amino acid (EAA). It's very common knowledge that too much EAAs will kill a neuron in a heartbeat. And some neurons are more susceptible than others. Furthermore, children's brain cells are more likely to die from EAAs than those of adults. These are all undisputed facts.

Now, make up a worst-case scenario. Let's say our children are consuming large quantities of something harmful. The people who make the chemical – no surprise – tell us over and over that it's safe. So the children still take it, and don't seem to have any obvious effects from it. So we let it go. But, in this worst of all cases, the ill effects don't show up until much later in life. (Like Thalidomide. Just because you don't see problems right away, doesn't mean they're not there.) Meanwhile, the problem it does causes makes the children take even more of it, which perpetuates the whole ugly mess.

That's a bad situation. Unfortunately, it's not fiction, but applies to us. This is what we know. Published studies with laboratory animals very clearly show that simply eating aspartame causes brain cell death in the hypothalamus. The immature nervous system is particularly susceptible.

If you kill your hypothalamus, what happens? You don't shake with motor problems or get numb from sensory problems. Among a host of other things, the hypothalamus controls feeding behavior. Furthermore, in a recent issue of *Neurotoxicology*, Dr. Olney pointed out that animals don't show the effects of hypothalamic damage right away. It surfaces later in life. These problems include obesity, alterations in the onset of puberty, and infertility. Do these problems sound familiar to you?

Go back to that worst-case scenario. Kids drink diet drinks with aspartame. We know this destroys cells in the area that helps control weight. Kids with weight problems naturally think, "Well, I should drink diet sodas then." The studies I mentioned were done in mice and monkeys, but humans are even more sensitive to EAA toxicity – approximately 5 times more sensitive.

"But the food company says it's safe!" That may be, but you must be skeptical of anything a used car salesman says about the car he's trying to convince you to buy. Here's a case in point. The industry's own research showed early on that there were no ill effects in monkeys from exposure to an EAA (from Reynolds and colleagues, see Appendix). Great. And this is what you will hear from manufacturers.

But they left out a small detail. The animals were kept anesthetized during the experiment. And the kind of anesthesia they used, we now know, specifically blocks the path through which this chemical kills your hypothalamus cells. No wonder they didn't see any problems in the monkeys. Damage by EAAs such as aspartate and glutamate is prevented by the experimental setup. So if your children are under *phencyclidine anesthesia* while they drink their NutraSweet soft drinks, I'd say they're safe. Otherwise, maybe they should have milk, water, or juice. But that's just me.

Listen, this is a hornet's nest. Consumer groups, doctors, and researchers are up in arms over the fact that there are 90 known dangerous side effects of aspartame. 90. They point out that well over half of the FDA complaints come from aspartame products. There's even talk of an "Aspartame Disease" (make sure to visit website references in the Appendix: "Aspartame").

The NutraSweet people say it's nothing – and have been saying that from day 1. But, you and I have had this lesson beaten into us over and over – corporations do not have a soul. Their survival depends on profits. Tobacco companies knowingly sold addictive carcinogens. Ford knew in 1989 about the danger of rollover in its SUVs and simply told people to deflate their tires to 26 psi. Pacific Gas & Electric allegedly dumped their alleged chromium into the alleged drinking water and told the alleged people it was allegedly safe. The list is shamefully long. How many examples do we need? The NutraSweet people will say their product is safe, whether it is or not.

The way NutraSweet got approved by the FDA in the first place is a mini-series docu-drama waiting to happen. The company that makes it, J. D. Searle, first applied for approval back in 1973. The independent board of scientists looked at all the data and could not conclude that it was safe.

In 1974, however, it was approved for restricted use in dry form. Independent scientists raised a red flag. An FDA investigation was launched to scrutinize Searle's data. They found that Searle's own research showed that, of the 7 infant monkeys given aspartame in their milk, 1 died and 5 developed grand mal seizures.

By 1977, the U.S. Attorney's office received a formal request from the FDA to investigate Searle for making false claims and concealing such harmful evidence. This office, though, did not even act on the complaint and the statute of limitations on the investigation ran out. Case dropped.

In 1979, the FDA established a Public Board of Inquiry to investigate NutraSweet safety issues. They determined that there was no "proof of reasonable certainty that aspartame is safe for use as a food additive." It's those darn tumors again.

Thumbs down.

Now go to 1981. The day after Ronald Reagan took office, Searle reapplied to the FDA for approval of aspartame (with no new data) because they felt that this new administration would be more business-friendly. This wasn't a guess. They knew it because they were on the inside track. Donald Rumsfeld was on Reagan's transition team. Donald Rumsfeld also happened to be the C.E.O. of J. D. Searle. Hmm.

So a new FDA head, Arthur Hull Hayes, and an entire new advisory panel were put in place for a re-try. Once again, the in-house FDA panel advised against approval. However, in 1981, Arthur Hull Hayes "overrules the Public Board of Inquiry, ignores the recommendations of his own internal FDA team, and approves NutraSweet for dry products" (see www.swankin-turner.com/aspartame/hist.html).

Meanwhile, the National Soft Drink Association lobbied the FDA not to approve NutraSweet. They opposed it because when aspartame gets above 86 degrees F, it breaks down into a common poison known as free methanol (wood alcohol). Your body, as you know, is normally 98.6F. Methanol is a problem because it breaks down into formic acid (normally used to strip off epoxy) and formaldehyde (the embalming fluid). This means that every time you cook up your sugar free Jell-O or put that little blue packet in your hot tea or coffee, you could be getting more than you bargained for.

Despite these concerns, Hayes granted FDA approval for the use of aspartame in carbonated beverages in 1983. Within 4 months, he left the FDA and took a position as a consultant in Searle's public relations firm. This is how the FDA approved aspartame.

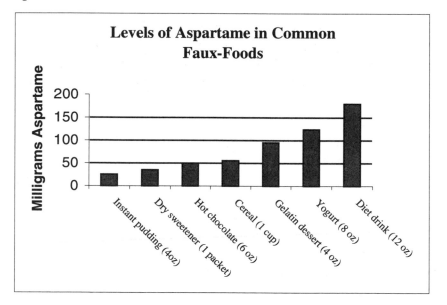

Like I said, this is a hornet's nest. But all of it is resolved when you follow the simple rule: if it ain't food, don't eat it. And let me tell you, aspartame ain't food. While the jury is out on this, don't let your children drink or eat or touch aspartame. Let someone else debate the fine points of biochemical pathways and government regulations. As far as these chemicals are concerned, it's dangerous until proven safe, not safe until proven dangerous. The possibility that your child can suffer long-term damage isn't worth a diet cola – no matter how much they whine, no matter how cool it looks on the ads, no matter how much some C.E.O. bobs his head while he's telling you it's safe.

Faux-Foods Quiz: A test for spies

This one's a gimmie-putt. If you can't guess it, you probably didn't grow up in this country. In fact, the Secret Service uses this as a litmus test to tell whether a possible spy is really on our side. Picture five guys in Humphrey Bogart trench coats glowering over the sweating individual in the center of a smoke-filled room. "Alright, *comrade*, what's this!"Then they read him the ingredients below and just hope he slips, as they all do, and says Snickers bar or something.

Ingredients

Peanuts, corn syrup solids,sugar, soy protein, fully hydrogenated rapeseed and soybean oils, salt, mono and di-glycerides, molasses, niacinamide, folic acid, pyridoxine hydrochloride, magnesium oxide, zinc oxide, ferric orthophosphate, copper sulfate.

Hint

The reason I added this is because I was completely floored by the incredible length of this list of stuff. Isn't zinc oxide usually found in diaper rash ointment?Life doesn't have to be this weird. Smuckers makes the same product. Look at their ingredients. There's only one thing in the entire list and, if pressed by the Secret Service, 99% of Vice Presidents surveyed would be able to spell it.

PUT THIS DIET INTO ACTION

·

10

The Specifics: Breakfast, Lunch, and Dinner

For mom it was different.
She came to live with us in France for a few months with no expectations about losing weight. She just wanted to love her food for a change before going back home to dig herself into yet another diet. So it was quite a shock when she realized she had gained nothing on the French diet – despite how decadent she had been. What an additional shock to realize that she had dropped 4 dress sizes!

But you, the reader, aren't unaware that you're trying to lose weight. And you've probably noticed that we aren't in France. So we have to deal with a culture that pushes low fat, high sugar foods at us, tells us to eat, eat, eat, and restaurants that make you hurry, hurry, hurry, etc., etc., etc. We have to be able to apply this diet in our lives.

When making this diet work for us, we need to have markers so we can see how we're doing. The most obvious measure is your weight. I don't want you to weight yourself everyday because, first of all, weight fluctuates a lot over the short term. It's only the long-term weight reduction that matters for us anyway. So just to get a sense of what's happening to you, weigh yourself only once per week. The point of this diet is to love your food. The point of this diet is to be healthy. The point of this diet is to develop a nutritious way of life. The pounds will fall.

Yes, I know. The very reason you're here is to lose weight. But a better indication of how you are doing on the diet is how often you eat. Here's a rule to follow: eat at meal times. Don't eat when it's not mealtime. Pretty straightforward.

Our bodies have been conditioned to snack and snack and snack just to make it from 8:00 to 12:00. But you don't have to be brimming with food to have your cravings go away for the entire morning. In fact, "stuffed" should never happen in this diet.

Add fat back into your diet and you'll be satisfied longer after breakfast. This frees you from having to nibble at 10:30. The same is true for the time between lunch and dinner. So I want you to note when you eat between meals. Then, after you've added fat to your diet, note when you make it to lunch without craving a snack. That's your goal. Once you reset your body's expectations, it becomes a natural part of you and no effort at all to keep from munching your way through the morning.

Now let's look at the specific situations during the day: breakfast, lunch, and dinner.

Breakfast

Hopefully you aren't eating breakfast at work, and hopefully you aren't on the road. Those cases can be handled as exceptions, but let's take the normal everyday case, when you're hopping up the hallway, pulling on you socks with one hand, and eating with the other. You have some choices here, but I'll put down my recommendations in the order you should try.

Before I start, though, I want you to pay attention to what time you eat breakfast. Then see what time during the day you get hungry. Not when you *want to eat* because someone evil has brought a dozen pudding-filled fudged-covered doughnuts into the office. Practice listening to your body and write down the time when you actually feel hungry.

Because the breakfast I recommend quiets your cravings, you will soon find yourself at lunchtime (and sometimes beyond lunch) without having needed a single snack along the way. Because you will be satisfied until lunch, you have already begun to eat less food.

First, buy some whole-milk yogurt. Stonyfield makes a good vanilla yogurt with cream on the top (you stir this in). But don't get the single serving size. The American "single serving" portions are simply too large, approximately 2 – 3 times as large as the French give for a single serving. So buy the largest container they have – the tub – and then dip out about 3 heaping tablespoons into a small dish.

Remember, exact amounts are not critical here: 2 tablespoons of yogurt, 4 tablespoons, whatever. No one could spell out a single diet that works for every person, and you shouldn't look to one-size-fits-all diets either. I am giving you general guidelines inside which you fill out the details that work for you personally.

When dipping out the yogurt, always use a clean spoon. Never lick off the spoon and then put it back into the container for more. That way you don't introduce your own little flavor into your yogurt. It also keeps it from developing other bacterial growths.

Several people have written me and said that they love mixing granola with the yogurt to make a delicious and substantial breakfast. That's a great suggestion. In either case, eat in small bites. I have a trick I use to help remember – focus on enjoying it. Weird. Our normal attitude disregards something so trivial as "enjoying your food." But if you have the stance that you are going to sit down and enjoy it, you'll take your time, eat smaller bites, and make it last longer.

If you like cereal in the morning, get a reasonable one – not frosted, chocolate-covered sugar bombs. I have raisin bran, but there are a hundred decent cereals that aren't loaded up with sugar. Avoid sugar cereals like the plague, because they increase your taste for sugar and encourage you to want more and more.

Putting fruit in your cereal is a good idea, too. I use a banana, but anything else will be fine. Use whole milk. Eat slowly. This is real easy stuff.

So. In the morning, eat your cereal or toast or whatever you have. If you are drinking low fat or no fat milk, you need to slowly work your tastes up the ladder to whole milk (see chapter: "Train Your Brain"). For the advanced course, for tough-guy Rambo commando types, follow the advice I mentioned at the beginning. Put a few tablespoons of cream in with your cereal. Now, if you have been drinking 1% milk forever, you will have to work up to the cream scenario. But, actually, this should be your goal. After you become comfortable with whole milk on your cereal, add just a small amount of cream. Man, it's good.

By the time you reach this level, the small amount of milk fat will take you through lunch and you will not be ravenous for anything in the vending machine. More importantly, you will be on your way to your target weight.

If you like to have a bagel in the morning – either at home or at the bagel shop on the way into work – that's no problem either. Have normal cream cheese (low fat cream cheese is not normal) or regular butter on it. Avoid jelly. Also, you must force yourself to take your time. I know how easily that bagel wads up into our cheek pockets. Eat one small bite at a time and finish it before putting another bite in. Start 30 seconds earlier if you have to. This is about you and your weight, you and your health. You'll get more pleasure out of your food and your body will get more nutrients out of it as well. You will be satisfied longer and you will begin to drop weight without even realizing what you have just accomplished.

Sometimes I'm just not hungry for breakfast. Especially when I've had a largish dinner the night before, or eaten late in the evening for some reason. My American training slips into my head and, sounding much like Charlie Brown's teacher, says, "Breakfast is the most important meal of the day." I agree with this, especially for children. My rule for myself, though, is this: if you're hungry, eat. If you're not hungry, don't eat. If I'm still satisfied from the last night's supper, I just wait until lunch. No problem.

But if you feel the need to have breakfast, or that you might get hungry later if you don't, have a touch of the whole-milk yogurt or a couple of nuts. Three tablespoons of creamy yumminess or 4 oily Brazil nuts isn't going to hurt anything.

That's it. Remember to note when you eat, and when during the day you get hungry again. The first few days will be hardest because your body is used to a certain *quantity*, and you will be re-training it on *quality*.

Lunch

Lunch is a tough meal, because there is such a range of eating routines during the middle of the day. Some people go out, some bring the brown bag, some stay home and graze through the fridge. If you go out for lunch, I'm going to refer you to the chapter on "The Plan: How to Eat." There I talk about dealing with the Paul Bunyan-sized troughs they serve you, the eat-pay-then-gettouta-my-restaurant attitude of many places, and the kinds of solutions for you to use.

Briefly, when eating out, I find that the appetizer portions often provide plenty. This is true as long as you eat slowly. So get a smaller portion whenever you can. Cut your serving into small pieces. Put your fork down between bites. Enjoy your food. If you do these things, the huge portion sizes will be too much for you to eat. Finally, listen to your body. When you're satisfied, stop eating.

As for the food itself, if you have soup, don't be afraid of the cream-based ones. If you have a salad, have it with lots of goodies: with ham, some boiled egg, carrots, croutons. Be sure to get a wide variety of food types in there. Salads are great foods, not because they're a low-cal rabbit food, but because they have a ton of nutrients you need. When you pick out a dressing for your salad, get something normal. Don't get the low-cal vinaigrette, or the fat free ranch. The Caesar or Bleu Cheese dressings are great. A favorite of mine is to just drench it in olive oil and a splash of balsamic vinegar. Simple.

The reason this is so important for you is that you can't even absorb the nutrients in your the salad if you eat it with fat free dressing. Also, on a more practical level, this makes the lettuce and the other veggies last longer through the afternoon.

It's a good idea to have a cup of coffee after lunch (or tea if coffee makes you too jittery). If you have time at the table, finish off your meal with it. Otherwise, stop by the coffee shop and have a small one. This is good for a couple of reasons. First, obviously, it takes that warm fuzzy blanket off your brain so you can think from 1:30 – 3:00. But it also finishes the meal in a way that helps carry you through the afternoon.

Whether coffee is important to diet, to digestion, or irrelevant to everything is unclear. But the French consider it an important part of the end of the meal. I wouldn't be surprised if some longitudinal study someday determined that coffee increased your body's metabolism of the food just eaten. I don't think anyone has looked to see whether coffee has a beneficial effect on digestion and weight, in the context of the French meal. So have a coffee as a finishing touch.

The final thing you need to do is the icing on the cake. After you have gone shopping and gotten some decadent cheeses, take a couple of healthy pieces with you to work. After lunch, eat a small one like a piece of fine candy. Let it "melt in your mouth" like butter. Have 1 or 2 nuggets each day after lunch. This satisfies your hunger, all the way to dinner.

Something else I do is carry a bar of the richest darkest chocolate I can find and keep it in my desk (Lindt makes a pretty good one, but there are plenty of others). To end my lunch, I eat one square, in little bites. Again, not chewing it up, but letting it melt so that I can enjoy it longer. Note: people can be fanatics about their chocolate. I want you to upgrade your chocolates to those that have as little sugar in them as possible, i.e., dark chocolate. Remember, "milk chocolate" is a euphemism for "more sugar and fillers added." You may have to make the switch gradually to get used to the new tastes. But it's worth it.

Attention Chocolate Lovers

Dr. Andrew Weil reported in his most recent book that certain kinds of chocolate have cocoa butter, which "have a beneficial effect on the serum lipid profile." So not only does it taste good, but it's good for you too. Remember, the best stuff is the rich, dark, high-quality chocolate. Enjoy.

This is important. The last parts of your lunch – the cheese nugget, the small chocolate piece, and the coffee – are all wonderful additions. But they also do a very important thing, as a bonus. They complete the meal and leave you satisfied throughout the day. Here's the point. Plan on eating an amount that will leave you needing a bit more after you are done. Then have the cheese finish, the chocolate piece, and the coffee to cap it off.

Dinner

Dinner can be extremely hectic. But you want to have good food for your family, not to mention yourself. Here's the problem. Unless you are a stay-at-home person, you generally don't have the stamina to cook something cool and fancy every night. Here's the solution. You don't have to. I'll give you some example recipes later that are easy to make and fit squarely within the spirit of the French diet.

First, the rules.

1. No prepackaged pig-in-a-blanket, pop-it-out-of-the-freezer foods. If you have to use this as an emergency, only do it once per week. Once. Be strong.

2. No snacky junk from a bag. No cheese puffs. If you want a snack, have a bit of yogurt, one or two unsalted nuts (eat them slowly), cheese, a hard-boiled egg, or a piece of fruit. Remember, always eat what you know. If you can't identify it as coming from a plant or animal, don't eat it.
3. Read the section on habits and follow those suggestions about your eating style and pace.
4. Variety is key.

One of the most important lessons of the French diet is that too much of anything is too much. So for dinners and lunches, serve plenty of variety. One way to think about this is to have a lot of colors. Salmon, green beans, and rice are excellent. Baked chicken, yellow squash, and mashed potatoes are wonderful. Grilled red peppers, asparagus, and lean pork chops …. You get the picture. Have some veggies, a meat, and some bread or rice. At a very fundamental level, it's true that you are what you eat. Balance in equals balance out.

You soon find that you'll have leftovers more and more often as you "downshift" the amounts you and your family eat. They'll just eat less food. So, start by making your meals from the recipe list provided. From there, you can decide how many nights per week you are comfortable cooking, when you should dip into the dim recesses of your refrigerator and pull out leftovers, and when you should just have snacky suppers.

As for vegetables, my French friends have told me that this represents a key difference between the French and American diets. The French have a "culture of vegetables." On the other hand, the American vegetable is … the potato. Americans eat them baked, mashed, as French fries, tater tots, and tater skins. They could eat them in a boat, they could eat them with a goat, they could eat them in the rain, they could eat them on a train.

Of course there's nothing wrong with potatoes. I love them. But there is something wrong with relying too heavily on only one type of vegetable. We don't eat other vegetables in quite the same way, because most Americans generally grow up seeing veggies as gross. There's no such thing as broccoli nuggets or an eggplant happy meal. You never see any squash-on-a-stick vendors at the county fare.

At home, then, we need to develop more vegetables in the foods we serve. I give specific examples in the recipes below. Moreover, re-introducing vegetables into your meals will be easier once you drop the fear of fat. Cooking with olive oil, butter, nuts, etc., makes them taste much better. Good, even.

The Reader Replies: Debbie

My own thoughts about this diet, which I am trying to follow.... The hard part for me is taking care of a 3-month-old and a 5-year old here at home. I can sit and enjoy dinner without rushing off somewhere, but breakfast and lunch can be a challenge to get my food in before the baby needs me. So I just eat small bites as I go.

The other parts are easy – adding the cheese or yogurt – I LOVE the cream on top!!! It is like a treat – and the smaller portions keep me from eating too much. I can make it on most days until the next meal but sometimes, on a heavy nursing day, I do need a snack between meals. I generally stick with the nuts or cheese.

I have not weighed myself this week, but it seems like I am on a 1 - 2 lb per week loss. I like that. But there is definitely not a decrease in my milk supply, and the baby is happy and growing VERY well.

SO that is that.
Hope all else is well!
Debbie

After dinner, the French usually have a selection of cheeses. A large wooden platter comes by your table with a variety of soft, pungent, crumbly, mild, strong, goat, and cow cheeses to choose from. Two or three small wedges are selected and eaten starting from mild and going to strong. (The strong flavor would swamp the mild flavor, so the milder one is eaten first.) What does the cheese do? The French believe it helps digestion.

It's unfortunate that we don't have this tradition, because it's a great way to cap off the lunch or dinner. If you want to think mechanistically, this puts just a bit of milk fat on board to decrease cravings and allow you to make it to the next meal without having to snack. I believe that ending dinner with cheese is one reason why the French don't feel the need to eat a huge breakfast.

The snacky supper

We usually associate gourmet cooking with elaborate daylong sprees of basting and marinating and carefully constructing the bubbling masterpiece. But it doesn't have to be that way. You can have a brilliant meal without ever turning the oven on. The snacky supper is a perfect example. Go by the bakery and pick up a loaf of good bread. Sourdough is a favorite with us. At home, pour ¾ cup of olive oil (also known as Italian butter) into a bowl, sprinkle in some crushed red pepper, oregano, or other Italian seasonings. That's all.

On a separate plate, sprinkle on a bit of some salty cheese like Parmesan or Asiago. The bread is a marvelous vehicle for the oil. Sample it with oil only, or with some cheeses. Another addition is to have a small bowl for balsamic vinegar. Most of the time – because I don't feel like washing a million dishes – I just put the vinegar in the olive oil bowl itself. These two really work well with each other.

What you will notice is that you begin to develop distinctions you never dreamed of before. Olive oil has a great flavor, with subtle differences between the many varieties. You'd never understand this if you only cooked with it. In the Mediterranean, it's often just taken by the teaspoon, like a tasty medicine. So drench your salad or your bread in it.

TAKE SMALL BITES. Don't make me tell you again. Enjoy your food. Set your bread down while you are chewing so you don't end up rushing though it.

Along with the bread, add some fruit or vegetable nibbles. Red seedless grapes are my favorite because they're so easy and tasty. Get some olives (not from a can) or wedge off some tomatoes. Make all the pieces of this nibble-fest small and manageable in your mouth. If you like sardines, kippers, or tuna, have a bit of that with your bread, fruit, or veggie.

Speaking of fish, sardines make a great addition to your plate. Plus, they are rich in cancer-fighting oils. Have the ones packed in olive oil. Sometimes I eat them on a hearty cracker or piece of bread for lunch and that's all I need.

Some things were just meant for each other, drawn together by some cosmic gravitation: peaches and cream, peanut butter and jelly, etc. One of these natural pairs is walnuts and bleu cheese. Ei, yei, yei, it's good. The bleu cheese should be creamy, not crumbly. Put just a bit on a walnut, red wine at the ready, and eat half of it. We usually do this while we are playing some game at the table with our kids. (By the way, you can use Roquefort, too, but it's expensive. There's a great Finnish one called Midnight Blue that's both affordable and outstanding. You'll probably have to ask the person in the cheese section of the store to order it.) Supplement this yummy combo with something else to round out the meal. Try other cheeses, like Brie, with a good cracker. Or a smoked Gouda, which goes great with grapes or a little Dijon mustard. Practice, practice.

All these things are suggestions to add in as you need them. Start with the bread and oil and go from there. Talk about a nightmare for old-school American dieticians! Carbs and oil!

Faux-Foods Quiz: Fool me once, shame on you

Some people are gullible. It's true. But others are legitimately fooled by their senses. You can't fault them for that. For example, we have developed elegant sensory organs that are exquisitely sensitive to environmental toxins. Animals that ate poison things, died. Those that didn't, survived.

But this recognition of dietary good versus evil only applies to real food. Faux-foods are inventions, like Spandex, and can't be found walking around in nature or growing on a shrub. Our bodies have not been exposed to these before, and aren't set up to handle them. You just don't run into grazing herds of sorbitan monosterates and aluminum phosphates out on the savannah. It's not normal or natural. These words don't even come up on my spell checker. I'd have to look in the Merck manual just to find out what they are.

Here's the bottom line. We get schnookered by clever ads and the sugary tastes of foods. Of course, no one out of High School believes advertisements, really. But it's important to remember that good taste and clever ads don't make it good for you, especially when they're faux-foods.

Ingredients

Sugar, corn syrup, water, partially hydrogenated soybean oils, flour, dextrose, cocoa, eggs, soybean oil, caramel color, red 40, whey, baking soda, aluminum phosphate, sorbitan monosterate, polysorbate 60, mono and di-glycerides, salt, corn starch, sorbic acid, soy lecithin, natural and artificial flavors.

Hint

This kid-favorite has a rosy-cheeked little girl for its mascot. It's very popular and backsliding into this pit of faux-food iniquity can be pretty easy. I have less of a problem avoiding these, lately, just because they're so very sweet (Sugar and corn syrup as the first 2 ingredients weren't enough, so they threw in some dextrose later on). My sweet tooth has gotten more and more sensitive – see the chapter called "Train Your Brain."

11

The Shopping List

Okay. Let's go shopping.
Once we return from the supermarket we'll purge the refrigerator, but for now we should settle on the kinds of things to buy for this diet. These are things you should have in stock around the house.

Before we set off, though, have a snack. This is a good beginning to the diet I advocate. A bit of peanut butter on bread works well, especially with a glass of milk. Of course, I think peanut butter is a universal food and goes with almost anything (carrots, apples, bananas, you name it). If you don't like peanut butter, you can have a few nuts or a piece of fruit.

Here are snacks not to have. Don't have something low in fat, and don't have something high in sugar (which is what most low fat foods are). So don't plunge into that secret stash of M&M's or nibble on a rice cake on the way out the door. This won't work. You have to sit down and have just a bit of something yummy now, so that you don't later buy everything the Keebler elf has to offer. The point is simply to not be starving while you're out trolling the aisles for food.

The following sections list the things you want to have on hand in your house. Most of them are needed for the recipes that come later on.

A normal level of fat

Cheese is normal. Milk is normal. We have become so indoctrinated into believing that low fat products are healthy and slimming, that our concept of "normal" has warped into something strange.

When we look at the big picture, low fat products are only prominent in this country. And only in the last 30 years! Remember, this is when our obesity epidemic really got rolling. Before that, our weight and the levels of fat in our diet were more like everyone else's in the world.

The point is that low fat products are not normal, and neither is the low fat mentality toward health and weight. Forget the fact that it simply doesn't work, it's a ridiculous and deviant change in our diets, compared to every other culture.

So when I say to have normal milk, I mean milk – not something that has to be prefixed by a qualifier like "low fat." When I say to have normal butter, I mean butter – not something that requires a picture, a label, and an FDA approval sticker.

Dairy

Clearly, dairy is a staple of *The Fat Fallacy* diet. Let me point out that the cheeses below are ones you eat with other things. They go with the meal in some way: like Parmesan goes with spaghetti and Mozzarella goes in a salad or in your lasagna. You could eat them alone, and that's okay too, but they are better if eaten with other things. You'll see them in the recipes. But the cheeses to have with your bread, or just as nuggets of yumminess after the meal, are (alas) often not found in most normal American supermarkets. You may find them if you are lucky enough to have a grocer with a good cheese department. If not, you may have to visit a farmer's market. Here's the rule. Look for the creamy high fat cheeses like Brie and Bleu (there are a million out there, so keep sampling to find what you like).

Many people have been raised on low fat or no fat milk. I was too. However, once you introduce normal whole milk into your diet, you will need less to be satisfied. Once you see this solution work for you, it becomes like the keys you've been searching the house for, the one's that end up being right in the center of the kitchen table the entire time. It's so simple. It's just gotten overlooked completely.

1. Whole milk
2. Whole milk yogurt (cream on top)
3. Butter
4. Eggs
5. Cream
6. Sour cream
7. Whole milk Mozzarella cheese
8. Parmesan cheese

Frozen section

There's nothing "wrong" with prepackaged, frozen vegetables. Just like there's nothing "wrong" with trying to devise heroic measures to get them to taste good. But why would you? Maybe if you are making a gumbo one weekend you might need some frozen okra. Otherwise, get fresh with your veggies.

Most of the other prepackaged foods can be used as "emergency food," like chicken potpies or a frozen pizza if you can find ones that aren't filled with additives. But avoid these completely if you can. My advice is, if you're really compelled to eat these, only get one for the entire week so you will not backslide.

Speaking as a connoisseur of ice cream, this diet supports and encourages you to go for your pleasure. In real estate, the three most important factors are – in this order – Location, Location, Location. Here, it is Moderation, Moderation, Moderation. And the bonus prize is that, when you eat quality foods, this is no longer as hard as it sounds. So when you eat ice cream, do what I've advised for eating your meal, put it in a smaller container. Don't fill a soup bowl or casserole dish with it, and don't eat out of the bucket! Besides you only need 2 scoops, and it'll look sad and lonely in that big bowl. Find a small dish that 2 healthy scoops will fill up. Use that.

The other part of this diet to come back to is the rule, "if you don't know what it is, don't eat it." If you are brave, look at the ingredient list on the back of some of the foods in your freezer. If it weren't for the picture, you wouldn't have a clue what it was! For this reason, buy Breyers ice cream or some similar brand that has ingredients that Johnny can read. "Milk, mommy, it says milk." You've never heard Johnny say, "Partially hydrogenated polysorbate unsaturated Red #40, mommy, it says partially hydrogenated polysorbate unsaturated Red #40."

1. Breyers ice cream

(We tried to think of something else to buy in the frozen section, but just couldn't. I guess the point is … eat fresh foods!)

P.S. If you need whipped cream for something, get some cream, then whip it. It's easy. Don't get the Cool Whip – two of the first 3 ingredients are processed sugars. Look at the end of the pumpkin pie recipe for my version of whipped cream.

Veggies

Let me stay out of trouble first by saying, quite out loud, that I love my mother. It's true. I had a wonderful childhood and she did a great job cooking for me. Most of the things she made were oh so good, and I could go on for days-without-number talking about them. Okay. That said, the vegetables she served had surrendered and died long before they were done being cooked. That was just the tradition of cooking at the time.

Vegetables generally evoke the same longing in Americans as a grub in a log. Why is this? The first reason is the problem of cooking them too long. This drains their flavor and gives them the texture of soggy cereal that's been standing in your bowl over night. There aren't many kids who'll fight tooth and nail over limp veggies that dissolve into mush the moment they get in your mouth.

Cooking with butter and other oils

Don't hesitate to cook with these to make your foods taste great. But it's very important not to burn the butter or oil. This converts their fatty acids chains to their more heart-harmful by-products.

The second main reason comes from the fear of fat itself. If you are afraid of cooking with olive oil or butter or cream, it will be darn hard to make the vegetables taste good. Low fat/no fat vegetables are just low taste/no taste vegetables. This effectively discourages anyone from eating them. Ever. So don't be afraid to lightly cook your green beans in a skillet with a mixture of butter, olive oil, and garlic – fat, fat, and fat (but it's good fat, good fat, and good fat). You mustn't be afraid to hack up two or three veggies, slather them over with olive oil, salt, pepper, and oregano, and broil them for a quick 15 minutes. They're awesome. Squash soup sounds like a nightmare, but when it is made with cream, onions, and garlic, it's honestly more like a dream (see recipes below).

I'll give specific examples later, but here's the general rule to get your family to overcome the grub-in-the-log effect: lightly cook them so they are just this side of raw, and be sure to add something that makes them taste good.

1. Asparagus
2. Green beans
3. Red bell peppers
4. Broccoli
5. Squash
6. Eggplant
7. Cloves of garlic
8. Sweet onions
9. Bag-o-salad
10. A lemon
11. Tomatoes
12. Potatoes

By the way, don't get vegetables in a can. The only exceptions to this ironclad rule are beans, and tomatoes you use in sauces. These things are okay to buy canned, but everything else that purports to be a vegetable only sells you because of the pretty printed paper picture on the front. Unfortunately, what's inside also tastes like the pretty printed paper picture as well. Just get it fresh.

Bakery

One of the things Jesus actually said in his sermon on the mount was, "Blessed are those who live near a reasonable bread store, for they shall wear mysterious smiles on their faces to the end of their days." It must have been very windy just at that time, or maybe some medieval monk said, "Bread store. Bread store? That can't be right." And he left it out. The reason I'm certain it must have been said is because it's a universal truth, like E=MC^2. If you can pick up good fresh-baked bread daily, indeed thou art blessed and shall live to 92. Amen.

My advice on picking out bread is this. If it has plastic around it, if you have no idea how long it has been on the shelf, or if you are certain it would survive in a landfill as long as rubber tires and baby diapers, don't get it. Get the bread that was baked only a few hours ago. You'll like it better anyway.

1. Bread

P.S. Here are some helpful hints on your new-found bread fetish.

- Buy your bread fresh every day if you can.
- If you can't, or you have leftovers from the day before, revive it by rubbing it with a bit of water and warming it in the oven at 300 degrees for about 10 minutes.
- Don't refrigerate the bread. Just leave it out, wrapped in its paper bag on the cabinet.

Meats

Like veggies, the meats you make for your meals have to be choreographed. As for fresh salmon, I wouldn't freeze it, then thaw it later and expect it to chew easier than a rubber sandal. Chicken has to be eaten right away or frozen. Pork chop filets are great, too, because you can buy a million of them and stick sets of 4 (if there are 4 people in your family) into a zip-lock in the freezer. Then when you want to eat them, just thaw them out and voilá! Ready to cook. Polish sausage, on the other hand, has a shelf life up there with steel belted radials and Wonder Bread.

Most of the meat recipes I show take no time to put together. Simplicity is the key to sanity.

1. Salmon filet
2. Catfish filet
3. Chicken, whole or in pieces (skin on!)
4. Pork chop filets
5. Polish or Italian sausage
6. Rump roast for a rare treat

7. Sardines, kippers, or tuna

P.S. Some people don't get into sardines, with their little body's packed in there like, well, sardines. If you don't mind them, they are an incredible element of one of those snacky suppers you have, and super healthy too. Just put them on a small piece of bread. Kippers are a good replacement if the sardines are too salty for you.

Which meats to eat

This is the French diet. So we are going to eat (in most ways) like the French. Refer to the section above on comparing food pyramids of the world. The least healthy culture chosen (ours) has the highest recommended levels of red meats.

Coincidence? Maybe, but I'm going with the populations that don't have all our heart problems.

- **In *The Fat Fallacy* diet, limit red meat consumption to approximately 1 time per certified blue moon, or once every other week, whichever comes first.**

- **Here's the hierarchy: Eat mostly fish, then chicken, then *lean* pork, then red meats.**

Other stuff

Some of the things in this section are helpers for meals, but many of them are for snacks. Again, make snacks something you understand, like unsalted nuts: almonds, cashews, Brazil nuts, pecans, walnuts, etc. Another bonus of nuts is that they are high in oils, so only a few are needed to satisfy your hunger.

Keep fresh fruits around. Nothing is easier than slicing up a pear to have at the end of a meal, or pulling off some orange pieces. Need snacks for a long drive? Dried fruits and grapes are great for this. Using these things to satisfy your sweet tooth allows you to have something healthy without overindulging in processed sugars.

As for your meal, I'm going to tell you to drink wine. Think about wine as a food to be taken at meal times like a vitamin (vitamin W). A beer works the same way (especially on a hot day), but wine is better for you and doesn't fill you up as much. Remember, we're not over-indulging in food, and we're not over-indulging in wine.

1. Walnuts
2. Brazil nuts
3. Unbelievably virgin olive oil
4. Balsamic vinegar
5. Oregano
6. Crushed red pepper
7. Canned white beans
8. Canned black beans
9. Canned field peas
10. A wine you like (not a sweet wine, preferably red)
11. Olives (not from a can)
12. Dried cranberries, cherries, raisins, etc.
13. Pears, plums, bananas, oranges, etc.
14. Whole wheat crackers (no additives, no sugar!)

What NOT to do

You know the "junk section" of the store? Yes, you know the junk section. It's the one with the chips and cookies and a broad range of orange puffy, gooey, crunchy things. Right, that one. You don't even need to swing by that aisle. Don't get me wrong. There is nothing on the planet wrong with chips made from 100% corn, for example. So read the label. If it's loaded with stuff that is bound to cause cancer in hapless laboratory mice, don't eat it.

There are salsas made with great ingredients. Those are fine for the occasional "snacky suppers" we have. But the other things are strictly off limits.

A long-term goal of this program is for you to reduce to zero the amount of snack foods you eat between meals. When you have "arrived," you will only eat at meal times.

Finally, don't drink soft drinks. This may be the hardest rule of all for some. First, it's just sugary chemicals – read the label. Second, even "diet drinks" have sweeteners in them and, aside from the issue of drinking aspartame (see section "Aspartame: A sweet toxin"), they condition your tastes to expect a certain amount of sugar. Once you get used to that level of sweetness, whether it comes from sugar or a chemical substitute, you begin to expect it in your meal, in your snacks, in everything. Luckily, however, the opposite is also true. If you cut down on your level of sugar intake, your tastes will grow to expect less in your meals and snacks. This is what you want.

If you need something to drink, drink something you know. Here are some exotic suggestions: orange juice, wine, water, milk, tea, coffee. Don't go into the soft drink section unless you are strong and can use the force, Obi-Wan, to keep from buying anything.

A good friend of mine surprised me when she said that her 3 daughters hated soft drinks. When I asked her why, she said that they never have them at home so the kids have no taste for them. "And you know what?" she added, "My kids have never had a cavity." I love talking to proud parents.

Faux-Foods Quiz: A little sugar, sweetie?

Why *are* American's so fat? A huge take-home message of *The Fat Fallacy* is that we have become paranoid of all fats. Our food makers respond by replacing them with tons of sugar. The four products below form a natural group – they just go together. But notice their ingredients. Every one of them has high-fructose corn syrup. Many of them combine this with sucrose and corn syrup because it just wasn't sweet enough. Given all that sugar, this product must be some kind of dessert. Right?

Wrong. That's what makes it so bad. Each of the products below is consumed at meal times. There's sugar in everything! These and most other faux-foods are eaten at lunch and dinner and disguise just how much *heavy sugar* you actually eat in every part of the meal.

Even in a stringent, rigorous fat free diet, if you eat sugar and sugar and sugar in your "food," you'll still get fat. This isn't rocket science.

Ingredients

1. Cucumber, high-fructose corn syrup, corn syrup, water, vinegar, mustard seed, salt, xanthan gum, spices, calcium chloride, alum, natural flavors, polysorbate 80, yellow 5.

2. Tomato concentrate, vinegar, high-fructose corn syrup, corn syrup, salt, spice, onion powder, natural flavoring.

3. Flour, water, high-fructose corn syrup, yeast, wheat glutanen, soybean oil, salt, soy flour, monocalcium phosphate, ammonium sulfate, calcium carbonate, mono and di-glycerides, ethoxylated mono and di-glycerides, calcium sulfate, datenin, sodium steryl lactylate, calcium dioxide, calcium iodate, diammonium phosphate, dicalcium phosphate, vinegar, enzymes, calcium proprionate, sorbic acid.

4. Water, high-fructose corn syrup, sucrose, caramel color, phosphoric acid, natural flavors, caffeine.

Hint
Define summer. This is it.

12

Meal Plans and Recipes

France lives in my memory.
It's like a wonderful dream you have just before you wake, when you drift in and out of that warm fuzzy space. Those are the dreams you remember, the ones you want to go back to sleep to find again. I've spoken to so many people that went to France and lost weight while eating sumptuous foods and returned to say, "How I wish I could eat those things here. Why can't I lose weight here?" They want to close their eyes and get back to loving their food, having fun, and losing weight.

Why can't we? This question has 2 meanings, and so it has 2 answers.

1. In the first sense of the question, why isn't our dietary culture set up so that we can succeed at losing weight? The main reason is that we've moved away from our

traditions. We've turned our heads so sharply toward the individual that we've ended up with our backs to the importance of the group and even the family. This mentality makes us more likely to eat alone in front of the TV, in the car, or at the office. Our culture has developed a very lonely element to it.

Another reason comes from the dietary blind alley we have taken for the past 30 years. For all the reasons stated in this book, we have invested our materials, our hearts, and our minds in the notion that you need to worry about the fat in your food. So all we see and hear and read supports eating more of the fat free foods. We end up eating tons of sugars and syrups in dinner foods that have been engineered to be low fat.

The last reason our culture has set us up for failure is precisely why America is so incredibly successful economically. We are a powerful nation of flexible entrepreneurs who work and move and groove to business's steady beat. The drive to make the buck and get ahead spins the hamster wheel at such a pace that there is little time for anything else. But hurrying through your food makes you fat. It's another irony: the very thing that makes us so successful also has its drawbacks – if you forget your core principles.

2. But consider the question from another angle. Why can't we adapt the French way of diet and health to ourselves? All it requires is a few modifications to take advantage of a philosophy that is mentally, physically, and psychologically pleasant. Once you think about it, there's no reason whatsoever we can't make the French diet work for us in America. We should be able to love our food, lose weight, and have a healthy heart in the process.

The French diet works. We can see that plainly enough just by the numbers of thin people there and fat people here. It also works for the scientific reasons I've mentioned already. So after showing it's validity, now we come to the practical end of things – the nuts and bolts of putting the French diet into play for you and your busy life. These recipes are laid out for

> ### Success?
>
> **Something to keep in mind as you frantically zoom through your life to get ahead:**
>
> **Even if you win the rat race, you're still a rat.**

people with hectic lives: for people who work, come home, and face making a healthy meal for their family. But because they are so simple to fix, they work just as well for anyone.

I want to point out that the meals and recipes you will see here are not fancy. Perhaps you might think that, because this is the "French diet," you would read about many an exotic flambé to fix or soufflé to whip up. Those are great to do, and there are plenty of cookbooks out there for them. But I'm going to start by giving you meals and recipes you can apply to your daily life. It's just good food, but I could add an é on the end if you'd like.

Taking our current lifestyle into account, I've divided the recipes into quick and easy *Weekday meals* and *Weekend meals* that require more time. You can't just come home from work and pop in a lasagna worth eating. You can't whip up a gumbo you can be proud of in 10 minutes. Those meals are wonderful, but need to be done on the weekend when you have more than 5 minutes and 34 seconds to breeze in, make dinner, fight the nightly fires, handle the children, straight up a bit, and at least make eye-contact with your family.

As for the Weekday meals, you'll find no heroic bastings or bubblings to do. Like I said, it's all just good, healthy foods. Notice too, that balance is built in to these meal plans, and so they are ready to go just as they're laid out.

Remember to improvise. Follow the dotted lines I lay out at first, and then have fun and tweak them into shape whenever you see a particularly yummy addition. If you follow the rule of thumb, and always taste as you go, you'll slowly develop excellent foods. Like any good meal, you'll find the desserts at the very end. But in this case, it's perfectly okay to skip down to those before you read all the mealtime recipes.

Weekday meals

Salmon filets, broiled potatoes, and asparagus Parmesan

This is a great dinner because it's so easy, but looks like you actually did something time-consuming and elaborate. It takes almost no time to fix because everything is done right in the broiler. And it is one of the healthiest dinners I can imagine.

You'll need:
>Salmon filet(s) large enough for everyone (~1/3 lb per person)
>One medium/small potato per person
>A handful of young thin asparagus spears (about 4-5 per person)
>
>1 lemon
>1 onion
>Salt
>Pepper
>Thyme
>Oregano
>Rosemary
>Olive oil
>Butter
>Parmesan cheese

Salmon filet.
- Take it out of the paper and rinse it in cold water. Lay aluminum foil on the counter and set the filet on it, skin-

side down. Rub over with generous portions of olive oil. Sprinkle with salt, pepper, and thyme (doing it in this order will make the herbs and spices stick to the oil and then cook into the fish). Cut the onion into thin slices. How thin depends on how much you like cooked onion. Set them end to end on top of the fish. Rub just a bit more of the olive oil on the top of the onion. Now take half a lemon and squeeze the juice onto the top of the whole thing. Now cut the other half of the lemon into a few slices and put them on top of the onion.

- Here's the trick. Put aluminum foil in a baking pan, and then set it upside-down on the fish. Now flip the whole thing over and throw away the first piece of foil. The skin faces upward. The onion and lemon slices will be on bottom with the oil. This makes the moistest salmon you have ever put in your mouth!

- Bake at 350 for only 25 minutes (this depends on how well your oven holds its heat). Test the fish with a fork at its thickest part after the timer has gone off. You'll smell it by this time. It should be only barely done. That's when the flavor is the best and the meat is the juiciest.

Broiled potatoes.
- Small red potatoes are best for this. But honestly, regular potatoes can be used just the same. Wash them first and leave the skin on. Cut them into small wedges, or quarters if you're using baby reds. Put them in a baking pan that you've covered with aluminum foil. Drizzle some olive oil over the top of them. You have to make sure all of the potatoes have oil on them. Sprinkle them over with the oregano, salt, and pepper. I'm not a salt fanatic, but I do find that potatoes require a lot of salt. See what you think when you make these.

- The olive oil coating is the key. That's what sizzles them to life on the plate and cooks in the spices without drying out the potatoes. So you may have to dredge them a bit in the run-off at the bottom of the pan to make sure they're covered. Sprinkle some rosemary on top.

- That's all. Now put them in the oven with the fish and wait until you smell them. When the fish comes out, broil the potatoes quickly until they turn brown and crispy on their edges.

Asparagus Parmesan.
- I know, I know. Asparagus. Yuck. I hated asparagus when I was a kid. But that's only because all they needed was a mild breeze and they would dissolve into Gerber baby mash, just waiting to be combined with Bartlett pears and strained beets.
- Even though there are many ways to mess these up, there are also ways to do them right. Here are the rules: never over-cook them, always have them with something rich and flavorful. If you are adventurous and have some time on your hands, make hollandaise. If not, here's an easy way to dress them up.
- First, pick the thinnest ones you can find. When you're ready for action, cut a full inch off of the bottoms and – just like the other recipes in this meal – set them in a baking pan lined with aluminum foil. (This is the meal I opt for when it is my turn to do dishes. You just wrap everything up in its foil afterward and throw it right away.)
- Spread the spears out like soldiers in a line, take some pats of butter and put them on their tops and bottoms. One top and bottom pat per 3 or 4 spears. Grate some Parmesan cheese generously over the top. Sprinkle them over with salt and pepper.
- These are also baked, then broiled. But be careful not to over cook them. If they come out like spaghetti al dente, you've gone too far. So hold off putting them in the oven until 10 minutes after the salmon goes in. They should bake for 10, broil for 5. You're done.

Sundried tomato pasta with vodka cream sauce and broccoli citron

I borrowed this pasta recipe from my dear friend Debbie. This is one of those recipes that sets a new standard for delicious. Although it's simple to throw together, it really ups the ante on flavor. But remember to eat it slowly. You'll want this one to last a long time. By the way, this makes a bunch. But the good part is that it's just as good reheated. Stir in a touch of milk and warm it up when you are having leftovers.

The broccoli adds a wonderful touch of greenery to the pasta and is super simple to make.

You'll need:
>   2/3 cup vodka
>   1 real good pinch of crushed red pepper
>   6 Tbsp butter
>   1 small box of penne pasta
>   1 cup tomatoes, blenderized
>   1 jar sundried tomatoes in oil
>   1 good handful mushrooms, sliced
>   1 cup whipping cream
>   1 cup fresh Parmesan

>   Enough broccoli for everyone
>   3 – 4 pats of butter
>   1 tsp olive oil
>   ½ lemon
>   Salt and pepper to taste

Sundried tomato pasta in 3 easy steps.
- Stir the amount of red pepper you choose (depending on your spice-tolerance) into the vodka, and begin the water boiling for the pasta. Don't forget to cook the pasta with some salt and olive oil.
- In a large saucepan, melt the butter over medium heat. Add in the vodka-pepper mixture, and bring it up to a boil. Add the blenderized tomatoes and cream. Return to

boil, lower heat, and let it work the flavors into each other at a simmer for 10 minutes.

- Chop the sundried tomatoes into small pieces. Sauté the mushrooms with the tomatoes in their own oil. Add to the sauce. When the pasta is done, add it to the whole batch, and mix in the Parmesan cheese. It's incredible.

Broccoli citron.

- Cut the florets as you like them and put them in a steamer.
- Steam them for about 10 minutes. When they're done, they will change from a dusty dark green (if they are fresh, which they should be), to a back-lit, vibrant green. You'll know what I mean when you see them. Take them off heat and uncover.
- Cut your pats of butter and olive oil and put them in a mixing bowl large enough to hold the broccoli. Then add in the salt and pepper, and squeeze in all the juice from the lemon.
- Throw in the steaming hot broccoli florets and turn them over so they get completely drenched. Keep doing this until the butter is melted. My children *ask* for this.

Cajun polish sausage, black beans, and yellow rice

This is a meal that is great because there are some secrets to doing it right. When I was in New Orleans at the neuroscience convention, we went to eat at a place called Mulatte's. When I got the polish sausage, I was thinking, how could they do anything different with this? It's just polish sausage, right? But when it came out I was stunned, instantly out of all the conversation at the table until I could taste this stuff and figure out what in the world they did to make it so good. Then, it hit me.

You'll need:

1 package polish sausage (feeds about 6)
1 can of black beans for every three persons

1 package of yellow rice

Worcestershire sauce
Olive oil
Cumin
Gumbo filé
Garlic salt
A small pat of butter

Polish sausage.

- First of all, don't get the low fat kind. Just regular polish sausage will do. It comes in a kind of almost-oval pack, so take it out and cut it in half at the bend. Then take that piece and cut it into inch-long segments. Now slice those longwise. You'll end up with a lot of pieces, but that's okay. Smaller bites are better. Save the other half of the original pack if you are only fixing the meal for a small number of people. Usually, the sausage is just fried in the pan as is, or with a little olive oil.
- But here's the secret. It's Worcestershire sauce. Just put it in the pan with the olive oil, cumin, and gumbo file and cook over medium-high heat. You may have to add some sauce, then add some more if the pan runs dry. Turn over the pieces a lot to make sure they all get seasoned.
- A couple of notes to remember. When cooking these sausages, cook them cut-side down first. If you start with the rounded skin-side down, the sausage will curl and you won't be able to brown the cut side easily afterward. So brown the other side first.
- Now for the health alert. This is a meal that is easy and yummy, but the sausage should be enjoyed no more than once per week.

Black beans.

- These come out of a can. Just pour them in the pan and heat them up. The way to get them to taste Caribbean is to add a sprinkle of cumin, a bit of garlic salt, and pepper.

All the while, after adding in what you think it needs, taste it again, then reapply more seasoning if you want.

Yellow rice.
- This comes in one of those long tube packages with its saffron spice packet. Because of some bizarre combination of chance and design, the flavors of black beans and sausage go great with the yellow rice. You can't avoid laws of nature like this. So just go with it.
- The instructions are easy. Just follow them and add a small pat of butter to enrich the tastiness of the rice. You can add salt and pepper to taste, but test it out first because the spice packet may be enough for you.

Pork chop filets, white beans, and bag-o-salad

I love good simple foods. And this meal is one of them. Pork chops: easy. White beans: out of a can. Bag-o-salad: open and serve. This is so easy. It's even nicer because you can buy the pork chops way in advance and just pop them in a zip-lock in the freezer. Again, this is a great set of healthy foods for people who work and need doable solutions to nightly meals without having to resort to frozen pig-in-the-blankets or some such.

You'll need:
Enough pork chop filets for everyone
1 can of white beans per 3 people
1 bag-o-salad

Lemon pepper
Garlic salt
Bay leaf
Cumin
Lemon
Small chopped tomato

Pork.

- It's really hard to mess these up. I don't want to jinx you, but really. All you do is take the pork chop filets and sprinkle each side with lemon pepper and garlic salt. Broil them in the oven until they're crispy. Voilá.

White beans.

- White beans are pretty plain by themselves. So you have to do a couple of things to make them lively. First put them in a small saucepan and add some salt, pepper, and cumin. Then throw in a bay leaf and about a tablespoon of olive oil. Chop a small tomato and add a squeeze of lemon too. Let this cook for about 15 minutes to get all the flavors mixed in. This will get you hooked on these beans. Note: I will not be held responsible for your newly developed white bean habit!

Bag-o-salad.

- You can get these at the grocery store with lettuce only, with different kinds of lettuce, with carrots in them, etc. It's great. One of the reasons I had always shunned salads was because of all the stuff you have to buy – one or two types lettuce, a bag of carrots, an entire cucumber. You only chop part of it up, because you only want a small salad to go with your meal. Then the leftover parts get filed into the back of the fridge. Realistically, however, they go straight into the "rot drawer." You leave them there for 2 weeks, open it up and say, "Ugghh!" Then you close it back up until you return to the store, clean out the mush with two fingers, and reload it with a new resolve to have salad in your life.
- That's why bag-o-salad is great. Just open it up, have the amount you want, and close it up afterwards. I like to add different goodies, depending on what I feel like that night. Sometimes I'll have walnuts and bleu cheese with it. Other times I'll throw in a slice of boiled egg or some olives. Then I put on a bit of normal salad dressing (like oil and vinegar, nothing non-fat).

Salmon patties, stunned spinach, and mashed potatoes

I had to argue with the editorial department to include this, because it frankly seemed too pedestrian to include in a book touting French food. Neither hoity, nor toity enough, you know. But I'm leaving it in because it's really as good as it gets. Number one, it's simple to make. It takes only about 20 minutes to make the potatoes, 15 minutes for the salmon patties, and 15 for the spinach. But mainly, it's great food. Next to Gumbo, this is my son Ben's favorite meal.

You'll need:

1 can of salmon for every 3 people
1 large bag of spinach for every 3 people
1 medium sized potato for every person

1 egg
Butter
Sour cream
1 good handful dried fruit pieces (raisins, cherries, etc.)
1 good handful pine nuts
Olive oil
Garlic salt
Salt
Pepper

Salmon patties.

- Canned salmon has to be separated from the bones that come along with it. Just put the meat into a separate bowl. Add an egg. Sprinkle with pepper and a little bit of salt (garlic salt if you have it). That's all. Mash them all together and form several sand dollar sized patties about a half an inch thick. Fry them in a skillet in olive oil over medium heat until they look brown and lightly crispy.
- Just a note on cooking. You have to let the bottom get crispy-firm before attempting to flip them. Otherwise the patty tends to fall apart.

Stunned spinach.

- You mustn't kill the spinach when it goes into the pan. Just stun it. I'll get to that in a minute. First, take off the stems and wash the spinach well to get off any remaining grit. Pat it dry.
- While you're doing that, throw the dried fruits into some warm water for them to soak.
- Put 2 – 3 tablespoons olive oil in a pan on medium high heat. Add a pile of the spinach because it will cook down to nothing in a hurry. Salt and pepper as you go.
- Be sure to rotate the pile all the time. You'll notice that the leaves on the bottom shrivel down like the witch in The Wizard of Oz. But here's the trick. You have to turn them off the bottom before they get all the way shriveled. They still need some snap and crunch to them.
- Take them off and put them on a side plate before they are even remotely wilted. Remember, stunned.
- While the spinach is recovering, pull out the berries from the water and dry them off. Throw them and the nuts into the pan with some more olive oil. Move them around as you heat them. When the nuts are browned and the berries begin to swell, turn off the heat. Then add back in the spinach to the mix. Toss them together, and then take them off. They're ready.

Mashed potatoes.

- I have to be honest. There's a problem with these potatoes. It's not the potatoes themselves, but now whenever I go back home for a visit, I am forced by family fiat to make mashed potatoes – a prisoner of this recipe. So don't even try this unless you want your family wagging around after you to make them every Thanksgiving and Christmas!
- Use red potatoes or brown ones, it doesn't matter. Wash them first. But – and here's a proprietary secret – don't take the skins off. The skins have tons of vitamins and they taste great! Slice the washed potatoes lengthwise into

halves, then quarters, then eighths. Boil them in salty water. When you can easily stick a fork through one of the larger pieces and it falls apart, strain them. Whether you like your potatoes more or less done is just a wonderful experiment waiting to happen.

- After draining, put them back into the large pan they were cooked in. Here's the magic (there are two parts to this, actually), and you have to just hold your breath and trust me on this one. Use 1 tablespoon of butter per person. If you expect to serve 4 people, well that makes a full half stick of butter. Breath in, breath out. It's all okay.

- Next, you need sour cream and a large spoon. I used to add milk to give them a nice smooth consistency, but now I just use sour cream. It's truly awesome. This is one of those things that I've never measured, so all I can tell you is to add a good bit (translation: about 1 tablespoon per person).

- Take a potato masher and mash everything up by hand. The potato masher makes the best potatoes because it leaves a flotsam of potato chunks in the mix. Experiment here. But don't taste them until you've added salt and pepper. For some reason, I find that I always need to add way more salt than I dream possible. When you do taste them, you'll know when you've added enough sour cream if you can just taste it in there. If not, get your spoon back out.

- With only a bit of practice these become the BPOTP in no time (that's the "Best Potatoes On The Planet"). Now you'll always have a job come Thanksgiving.

Bean Burrito

If you're ever in Atlanta, you have to go to Tortilla's. This is a hole in the wall, it only serves one thing, and you'll find as many tie-dyed dreadlocks as you will three-piece suits and soccer moms. You can get your bean burrito shaped like a taco, in a flour tortilla, or in a corn tortilla.

What has kept this eatery icon going for so long is that it's so incredibly good. When Dottie was pregnant with Grace, we went to Tortilla's 4 times per week. I kid you not. Some women go for ice cream or pickles, but Dottie had to have Tortilla's burritos. Grace is made of beans, Monterey Jack cheese, green chilies, and their unexplainably good Red Sauce. After I left Atlanta, I never really missed Braves baseball, the drenching summer rains, or terminally long commute times, but I couldn't wait to go back and get a bean and cheese burrito, extra cheese, and a green chili. Don't forget the beer.

After visiting my sister-in-law for Christmas, Dottie and I snuck off on our own for Tortilla's with three goals in mind:

1) To eat.
2) To get enough "to go" for another couple of days.
3) To taste for the ingredients to make it ourselves so we wouldn't get withdrawal symptoms after we went back home.

Below you'll find a pale comparison, I freely admit, but it's darn good anyway. Plus, this is something you can easily make in a crock-pot on a weekday, and it has lots of healthy goodies in it.

You'll Need:
    1 bag pinto beans
    1 – 2 Tbsp chili powder
    1 – 2 Tbsp salt
    3 bay leaves
    2 cloves garlic
    Flour tortillas
    1 good-sized wedge Monterey Jack cheese, grated
    Your favorite salsa
    Sour cream (the whole milk kind, you know)
    1 green chili (for the brave at heart)

Before you leave for work.

- Wash the pintos and throw them in a crock-pot filled with well-salted water. Just add the chili powder, garlic, and bay leaves. Now turn it on and leave.

When you come home.

- First of all, the house will smell incredible. Pull out a couple of the beans and test them for firmness. They should be just-soft.
- Take the tortillas out and put them on some aluminum foil. Wet a paper towel, place it over the top, and set it in the oven on a low heat to warm.
- Grate the cheese. Open the salsa and sour cream.
- If you're having chilies, put them in a pan in the oven on broil and turn them occasionally until the skin crinkles all over. Pull them out, peel away the meat, and test it to see how much heat you are prepared for.
- Now make your creation. You'll likely end up not putting enough beans in your burrito to start with. When this happens, I unroll it and then toss some more beans in, or just "top-it-off" without taking it all apart.
- It's the combination of the beans with the Jack Cheese makes this work. So don't be shy with the cheese. The sour cream and salsa don't hurt either.

Weekend meals

These meals take a bit more time to fix. But they're worth it. You can make them on an early Saturday or Sunday afternoon for supper, and then save the leftovers for warming up during the weekday.

Chicken with 40 cloves of garlic, just-done green beans, mashed potatoes with gravy

This is a great meal. Especially for a weekend. For us time-conscious, type-A, hustle and bustle Americans, the only thing keeping this from being a Monday-Friday meal is the fact that the chicken takes about 90 minutes to cook. If that's okay with your schedule, make it during the week. But we usually have the time on a "cookin" Saturday. Either way, you won't regret it. When that chicken falls apart and spills its aroma throughout your kitchen, you'll know that this is what heaven's chef serves to all the good little boys and girls – whenever they want.

You'll need:
>   1 medium whole chicken
>   1 medium/small potato per person
>   A large handful of green beans
>
>   1 rock hard head of garlic
>   1 onion
>   Salt
>   Pepper
>   Sage
>   Rosemary
>   Bay leaf
>   Olive oil
>   Butter
>   Sour cream
>   Sliced garlic

Baked Chicken.

- The set-up on this is super simple. Line a pan with aluminum foil and put the chicken in it. Rub it with plenty of olive oil and then sprinkle it over with salt and pepper. Take the garlic cloves – don't even peel the skin off – and tuck them under, in, and around the chicken. Put plenty of your herbs (rosemary, sage, and bay leaves) around.
- Cover it with foil. Cook it at 350 for 90 minutes. You'll smell it before it's done. Uncover and broil for the last 10 minutes to make the skin crispy.
- The baked garlic cloves in this are superb. If you have bread with the meal you can smear the garlic on it like butter!

Garlic green beans.

- Garrison Keillor said that rhubarb pie was one of the secrets to the good life. He's from Minnesota. Where I grew up, we thought rhubarb was a sticker bush. I have to say, though, since moving north of the Mason-Dixon, that I had rhubarb pie once and it was tremendous. What I would add to Mr. Keillor's trove of life's wonderful secrets is cooked garlic. Adding it to olive oil in a pan will make green beans a weekly staple.
- To begin, you have to rinse the beans and then snap the little ends off. Boil salty water, then add the beans. Let them boil for 5 minutes. Now here's a trick from Julia Child. After draining, rinse with cold water. Then drop them into a dry frying pan. Heat on high while you steadily move them around. The point? You evaporate off the water before you throw in the olive oil and garlic.
- Now just pour in olive oil (about a tablespoon), butter (one self-respecting pat), and the sliced garlic. Warm this on medium heat until it's melted and all mixed together.
- Make sure the garlic gets off the tops of the beans and down into the oil. Uncooked garlic is way too strong.
- Add salt and pepper. Sauté for only about 10 minutes. By the time the beans are just tender (you'll get to taste them

as they come along, a benefit of being the cook), the garlic will be just a bit browned or crispy. Watch the oil as you go, because it will be absorbed into the beans. Just drizzle in a bit more if you need to. Serve them hot.

Mashed potatoes and gravy.

- You can look above for the mashed potatoes recipe and use that. The secret here is the gravy.
- Take the drippings from the chicken pan and put this stock in a saucepan. You are essentially going to make a thin roux similar to what you'll do for the gumbo below. On medium heat, lightly sprinkle in about 3 tablespoons of flour, whisking it smooth as you go. You'll do this until it gets quite thick. Then just add about a quarter cup of water, whisking all the while, to make sure it stays smooth.
- Salt and pepper to taste. This gravy is dirt simple, but you can make it as thick you like it by varying how much water you follow it with. This goes on mashed potatoes like a cherry goes on a banana split. Perfect.

Tenderloin au Lait
with Mediterranean potatoes and roasted veggies

We bolted from the table as soon as we heard her scream. It was Grace. Something was dreadfully wrong. Dottie and I launched up the stairs to find our little girl, wailing on the bathroom floor. Her face in clear agony, her left hand clutched the base of her right pointer finger. Tears streamed down her frightened face.

"What is it!" we cried.

"I'm bleeding!"

It was true. There, high atop her outstretched victimized finger, was a tiny dome of blood – almost as large, but not quite, as a ladybug. I was so relieved that I made the common fatherly sin of chuckling at my daughter's misery.

"I'm *bleeding*!" she repeated even more emphatically for her dim parents, who clearly weren't tuned in to the desperation of this dire predicament. So I cleaned up my mirth for her as we cleaned up her finger. All the while, we talked about bleeding, giving blood for the Red Cross, and how blood-outside-your-body didn't always mean you were in pain. If you *are* in pain, it'll hurt. That's how you'll know.

I brought this up because we all have associations between food and yuckiness. If it's spoiled, it's bad. If milk is curdled, it's gross. But in this case, I'm going to ask you to suspend your beliefs – no screaming – because there will be curdled milk. It's not because it'll be left on your counter for 10 days in the sun, but because you simply simmer the tenderloin in it for 2 hours. Don't let this weird you out. You just blenderize it afterward to get the texture right. And it becomes the most exceptional gravy at the end. Moreover, the meat is so tender you won't even need a knife.

You'll need:
>   1 pork tenderloin
>   4 large potatoes
>   1 red bell pepper
>   1 small eggplant
>   1 Vidalia onion

For the tenderloin:
>   A sprinkle of salt and pepper
>   ¼ stick butter + 1 tsp olive oil
>   4 cups milk
>   2 pieces thyme
>   2 bay leaves
>   3 pieces parsley
>   4 garlic cloves, minced
>   Nutmeg, grated, as you like it

For the Mediterranean potatoes:
>   ¾ cup whole milk
>   ¼ cup heavy cream
>   2 cloves garlic, crushed
>   Salt and pepper

¼ tsp cinnamon (½ tsp if you like cinnamon)
½ tsp nutmeg

Roasted Veggies:
    Olive oil
    Oregano
    Salt
    Pepper

Tenderloin au Lait.
- This dish is so simple. I made it a weekend meal only because it takes about 2 ½ hours for it to work itself into melt-in-your-mouth status.

Prepare the meat.
- Take the tenderloin out of its package and strings. Rub it thoroughly with salt and pepper.
- Put the butter and oil in a pot over a medium high heat. Then seal in the juices of the tenderloin by searing all sides until just crispy brown.
- Discard the cooked butter when you are done.

Let it cook.
- Now just toss in all the milk and spices and let it simmer away for 2 hours. We've found that the sauce needs to cook down, so take the lid off after the first hour and let the aroma fill the house. After 2 hours, pull the herbs and meat out and blenderize the sauce. You can thicken it with flour if you need to.

Mediterranean potatoes.
- Sauté the garlic slowly in the milk, cream, and spices.
- Slice the potatoes very thinly.
- After you feel the garlic and spices have cooked all their flavors into the cream, turn the heat up to medium-high and add the potatoes.
- Cook these for 5 – 10 minutes. Careful turning them so they don't break.

- Then put them in a greased baking dish and bake at 350 for 1 hour. If the top isn't golden brown at the end, just broil it for a minute.

Roasted Veggies.
- Chop all veggies into small bite-sized pieces and lay into a pan lined with aluminum foil.
- Drizzle over with olive oil. Lots of olive oil. Be sure to dredge them in it so they don't dry out in the oven.
- Sprinkle them with salt, pepper, and oregano.
- Broil for about 15 minutes or until the edges begin to brown.

Note: This is a very good spring or summer recipe because you can get fresh herbs. This makes all the difference in the world. The old dry ones will work and, alas, I have to resort to them too at times. But if the stars have smiled on you and you live near a quality market with excellent herbs, get them. You won't regret it. By the way, this is also a good time to add a chilled dry white wine to your table.

<u>Lasagna</u>

This is honestly the best lasagna I've ever had. Dottie makes it and, although *she says* she's not Italian, I'm not so sure. I've tried many lasagna in search of the exception to the rule, but this one's the best.

You'll need:
<u>For the sauce:</u>
    1 lb spicy Italian sausage
    1 onion, chopped
    4 garlic cloves, minced
    1 large can whole tomatoes
    1 small can tomato sauce
    Salt and pepper to taste
    1 or 2 bay leaves

1 tsp oregano
1 tsp basil
1 pinch cayenne
½ cup red wine

For the Ricotta cheese mix:
1 16 oz container of Ricotta cheese (not low fat)
1 egg
¼ cup Parmesan cheese, grated
Salt and pepper to taste
1 tsp oregano

Mozzarella cheese
1 lb whole milk Mozzarella cheese, grated

Lasagna noodles

First, make the sauce.
- Cook the Italian sausage over medium heat with the chopped onions and minced garlic.
- After it's brown, add the whole tomatoes and tomato sauce right into the frying pan. Cut up the whole tomatoes into bite sized pieces.
- Add in all the spices. Throw in about a half-cup of red wine. Simmer for 10 minutes. Taste and adjust seasonings. When you think you've got it, let it sit and bubble on low heat for a while, because it only gets better as it cooks.
- Tasting is the key, if you are really going to evolve this sauce over time into a Zen state of Italian ambrosia.

While the sauce is bubbling its way into its various stages of perfection, make the Ricotta mix.
- Add the Ricotta, egg, Parmesan, salt, pepper, and oregano into a large mixing bowl.
- Use your own editorial license here. You may be reading this recipe and thinking, "¼ cup Parmesan? Only ¼ cup

Parmesan?" If so, throw in some more. Your whimsical creative impulses will evolve this recipe over time.

Grate the Mozzarella into a heap on a separate plate.

Boil 12 lasagna noodles in a pan of salty water and a good glug of olive oil.

Now build your creation in a standard lasagna pan.
- Place the pasta on the bottom layer.
- Spread about ⅓ of the Ricotta mix onto the pasta.
- Spread about ⅓ of the sauce on the Ricotta mix.
- Sprinkle about ⅓ of the Mozzarella onto the sauce.
- Repeat that process for the remaining ingredients.

Into the oven.
- Bake at 350 for 45 minutes. You'll smell it when it is getting close. When it's crisping a bit on the top and bubbling up on the sides (or you can't resist it any more) pull it out and allow another 30 minutes for it to cool and set up a bit.

This meal screams for a salad, fresh bread for sopping, and some red wine – the whole package. You'll notice that this ends up being a lot of food. So it's a great example of a meal that needs small portions. I agree, this is a tough one to restrain yourself on, but serve yourself a small enough piece so you know you'll have to come back for seconds. The smell will make your wayward hand stray to larger pieces, but be strong. Between the greens you have beforehand, the bread, and the pasta, you'll be surprised at how little you need to be satisfied. Remember to take your time with it. Trust me, it loves you too.

As you've noticed, this meal supports the rule to eat in courses whenever you can. The time when the lasagna is cooling is a perfect time to have your salad. After you're done and the lasagna is well cooled, have the main course and bread.

Authentic Louisiana Gumbo

Will Clower. It's not a Cajun name. Maybe a gumbo recipe would be more credible coming from someone named Lafayette "crawfish" Prud'homme. But this gumbo really is authentic.

Even though, it's true, I have no bayou water splashing through my veins, I managed to get some good recipes and sneak them back east after my sister married a certified, born and bred, crawdad-snatching, zydeco-stomping Cajun. I'm not sure how legal it is, exporting genuine Cajun recipe magic across state lines, so just keep this to yourself.

My son is a picky eater. He knows what he likes and, more importantly for him, he knows what he doesn't like. This gumbo falls into the first category, and has become his definition of great food. He told me he looked in the dictionary under "awesome!", "rockin!" and "dude!" to see if gumbo was in there. I guess there needs to be a dictionary for 13-year-olds. In fact, gumbo has become a reward item for him – a prize for good efforts and noble deeds benefiting humanity at large. However, we've had to draw the line at him bathing in gumbo or eating it for more than 2 meals per day.

You may notice below in the "You'll need" list that some of the items are a bit vague. I'll explain everything below. There's a bit of alchemy involved. After all, it is authentic.

You'll need:
>2 gallons water
>8 large chicken pieces, bones and skin still on them
>1 small handful salt
>3 – 4 bay leaves
>3 lb spicy sausage
>1 cup vegetable oil
>A little more than 1 cup flour
>2 large onions, finely chopped
>2 cloves garlic, minced
>¼ cup parsley
>1 – 2 stalks celery
>Red and black pepper to taste

Tabasco
Gumbo filé
Green onions, chopped

First make the stock.

- When you get the chicken, be sure to buy the parts with skin and bones still on them. This dramatically adds to the flavor you get on the other end. One result of the fat free frenzy is that people tend to just eat breast meat, and avoid legs and thighs. For the gumbo, you should include both. The darker meat is richer and, frankly, has a better flavor.
- Put them all into the water with the salt and bay leaves, bring it to a chummy sort of boil in a large gumbo pot. During the early part of the boiling you'll notice some whitish foam gooze bubbling on the top. Get a large spoon and ladle this out. It's yuck. The stock should boil along until the chicken meat falls off the bones, about an hour or so. In the end, your stock should have boiled down by about ¼, from 2 gallons to about 1½ gallons.

Make the sausage.

- There are a couple of options here. You'll have to play with them to see what works best for you (I always love it when I'm instructed to "play with my food").
- You can get the firm Andouille sausage that slices into small medallions and fry them up like that. They're generally very spicy, but it's really great when this flavor seeps into the broth of the gumbo.
- If you are not such a fan of spicy foods, you can also get the hot Italian sausage, which comes in the casing. Squeeze it out into the pan and chop it up as it cooks. Even though it says "spicy" Italian sausage, you'll be adding it to a vat of gumbo, so never you fear.
- Either way, you simply cook up the sausage and set it aside.

Remove the chicken from the bone.

- After the stock has cooked down by a quarter and the meat is falling off the bones before your very eyes, pull out the chicken and pull off the meat.
- Let it cool a bit first because it'll be quite hot. But be careful to remove all of the bones.
- Cover the chicken and set it aside with the sausage.

Do the roux.

- Roux is the elixir of life. Not many people know this, although I guess this book has let the cat out of the bag now. If you do this part of the recipe correctly, your gumbo will be triumphant! (Triumphant. No kidding, you just wait and see if you don't agree with that word at the end.)
- Get a 2-cup measuring container. Fill the first cup with vegetable oil. Now stir in some flour until it's smooth. Keep stirring in flour until the level gets up to 2 cups. You'll end up adding in much more than 1 cup of flour to the oil, because it all mixes in together.
- After the total beige mixture levels out at 2 cups, get a rubber spatula and scrape it into a frying pan over medium-high heat. You'll need a metal spatula to turn over the roux as it cooks.
- Here's what you're shooting for: chocolate. Not Hershey's milk chocolate, a rich dark chocolate. As the roux cooks and you turn it, it will go from an anemic pale, to milk chocolate, to a fine dark chocolate. Also note the texture. This will go from liquidy, to firmish and bubbly, to crumbly. When it gets to "crumbly dark chocolate," remember the aroma you smell. This means you have arrived at gumbo nirvana.
- Now for the alchemy. Watch out that you don't scorch the chocolate. Keep the roux just this side of burned. I can't tell you where that line is, young Jedi knight, so you'll have to use the force. Or maybe just be conservative to start with and take it off when it's crumbly and dark, but not yet burned.

Add the roux to the stock.

- Careful here. The chicken stock is water-based. The roux is oil-based. These two like each other as much as two irate alley cats in a shower.
- Take just enough roux to fit on your spatula and set it down into the pot, but not all the way down into the stock. Have the lid in the other hand because it's going to hiss and spit at you when the roux hits the water.
- After all the roux is in, boil it hard for 1 hour. Stir occasionally.

Finish the gumbo.

- After the roux and stock have boiled themselves into blended perfection, put in the chicken, sausage, vegetables, salt, pepper, gumbo filé, and Tabasco. Let these flavors simmer for another 20 minutes.
- You may notice that I did not specify any amounts for the salt, pepper, gumbo filé, and Tabasco. I want you to add these in as you taste. You'll get a feel for how much is enough. Remember, you are cooking in a vat, so you may need more than you think.
- Add the gumbo filé last. It gives it that "dirty" flavor that's the essence of Louisiana cooking. Add, taste, add, taste.
- When it's ready, chop some green onions to sprinkle on top.

Gumbo is served in a bowl, on a bed of rice. I dash some Tabasco in on top. But then I like it hot.

Squash Soup

The reason Ponce de Leon, that optimistic Spaniard, never found the famed Fountain of Youth wasn't for lack of trying. He was quite energetic. But it's a (very) little known fact that one day, after weeks of marching his men through the thickets of the pre-Disney Floridian forests, he came upon a clearing. Within the perfect grassy circle stood a well, raised on its knoll like a baptismal font prepared from the finest marble.

Sensing the completion of his quest and the validation of his sanity, he stumbled upward as the sun sliced through the primeval mists and the wind brushed back his long curly locks in a very Steven Speilbergian pose. He knew that the culmination of his work had been reached at last. He had finally found the fountain of youth. He would live forever. He stumbled to the top and reached the perfect smooth marble basin. Looking over its rounded edge, he couldn't believe his eyes. He lowered his hand, drank from its nectar, and wheeled about dramatically to his men.

"Wrong fountain," he yelled. "This one's squash soup."

Everyone groaned in unison. And the disappointed band tromped off into the waiting trees. If only he had known about beta-carotenes. These are found in abundance in yellow and orange vegetables and prevent cancer. This squash soup recipe, then, must have been what Ponce de Leon found so long ago and mistook as the work of juvenile native pranksters. It combines butternut squash with just enough creamy flavors to make sure your body can absorb the cancer-fighting carotenes and keep you ticking forever (your individual mileage may vary).

You'll need:
3 Tbsp olive oil
2 onions, chopped
½ tsp cinnamon
½ tsp coriander
About 2 ½ lbs butternut squash (acorn squash is good too)
3 – 4 cups chicken stock
1 cup half-n-half
4 pats butter
Salt and pepper to taste
Parmesan cheese, grated

To start.
- Cut the squash in half and remove the seeds. Peel away the outer skin, and then cut its meat into modest cubes.
- Heat the olive oil over medium-high heat. Add and sauté onions. Add in the spices, squash pieces, and stock. Bring to a boil, then reduce the heat until you achieve a cheery little simmer.

Next.
- Let it bubble away, covered, for about 20 minutes.
- At this point the squash should be done. Take the pieces out and blend in a food processor until smooth. Add them back to the pan, then add in the half-n-half and butter.
- Season it with salt and pepper. Taste. Depending on what you like, you could touch up the cinnamon flavor, too. Taste again.

At the table.
- Top this soup with a bit of grated Parmesan. Add in some good crunchy bread and it makes its own meal.

Desserts

Desserts. This is why we're on this planet. You can go to the highest mountain monastery and ask the squatting monk for the true meaning of life ... or you could just read along further (it's one of the added benefits of this book). The monk would look up at you with his very serene face and say, "Dessert, number one. And number two, good dessert. I never get really good dessert up here." Then he'd go back into his meditative trance. There you have it. And I don't even charge extra for this little bit of monkish wisdom.

A pie finishes the meal like a paycheck finishes the week. I need to emphasize that the pies, like all the desserts below, are to be treated with respect. No ravishing – unless, of course, you do it in little bites. The worst thing you can do for your diet is load up on too much dessert. Have your piece and love it too. Then walk away and live to eat another day.

Pumpkin Pie

Despite the fact that Dottie's pie has displaced my mom's pumpkin pie as the fairest in the land, she and Dottie still speak. Actually, mom has given up the old ways of cooking with sweetened condensed milk, and adopted this recipe. So much for that old saw about old dogs and new tricks.

This recipe makes 2 pies. Important: *The Fat Fallacy* diet considers small slices of pumpkin pie to be an important part of a balanced breakfast.

You'll need:
> 1 large can pumpkin (not pumpkin "mix")
> Whole milk
> 1 cup sugar
> 3 eggs
> 1 heaping tsp ground cinnamon
> 1 level tsp salt
> ½ tsp ground ginger
> ½ tsp ground cloves
> 1 package All-Ready Pie Crusts

Getting ready.
- Pour the can of pumpkin into a very large bowl.
- Fill that can with whole milk, pour it into the bowl, and mix until smooth.
- Add the sugar and eggs. Mix well.
- Take 1 cup of the mixture you just made and add: Cinnamon, salt, ginger, and cloves.
- Be sure to mix it around to get out any clumps of spices. When it's smooth, add it back to the main bowl.

Preparing the pie.
- Take the All-Ready Pie Crusts from the package (there should be two) and form each to the bottom of a pie pan, preferably one made of clay.
- Pour the mix into the crust.
- Bake at 425 for 10 minutes.
- Reduce to 350 for 45 minutes to an hour.
- You know it's done when you get your hot pads and jiggle it a little. The center will look like just-firm Jell-O.

Eating instructions.
- You have to let it cool a bit for it to firm up (about 2 hours). If you're in a hurry, put it in the refrigerator.
- When you can't stand it any more, here's what *not to do*. Do not mar it with a fake whipped cream.
- Because we all know that pumpkin pie screams for whipped cream, I'll give you the recipe. It's very easy.

Whipped cream.
- Take 1 pint of cream and add in 1 teaspoon vanilla, and 1 tablespoon sugar, then whip it. There's a trick though.
- You've got to do it in a very clean bowl or pan. If there are any residual oils, it will not fluff as well. We just put ours in a well-sealed Tupperware container and take turns shaking it until it thickens up (about 100 shakes or so). This is not the easiest method on the planet to whip cream, but it's a sort of family tradition.

Apple Pie

There's a problem with the pumpkin pie recipe above. Integrity and a healthy fear of lawsuits compel me to be straightforward with you from the outset. You really only find pumpkin around Thanksgiving. That's great for a month or so of the pumpkin-induced frenzy, but you're basically high and dry from January to October. Disclaimer done.

The apple pie, on the other hand, can be made any time. I know this because we have tested this theory, making it at many times of the year, just to make sure it's safe. Can't recommend something until it's well tested, you know.

This apple pie recipe makes 1 round pie from heaven. After it comes out of the oven and the angelic glow wears off, slice it fairly among the family. It comes with its own guardian angels to insure portion fairness.

You'll need:
>   5 lb bag Granny Smith apples, peeled and sliced
>   (no core, no seeds)
>   ¾ cup sugar
>   ¼ cup all purpose flour
>   1 tsp cinnamon
>   ½ tsp nutmeg
>   5 healthy pats butter
>   1 sprinkle sugar
>   All-Ready Pie Crust

Getting ready.
- After you peel and slice the bag of apples, put them in a large bowl.
- Mix the sugar, flour, cinnamon, and nutmeg in a separate bowl.
- Stir this mixture back in with the apples. Use a large wooden spoon to turn everything over and make sure all pieces are well covered.
- Important: lick fingers when done.

Assembling the pie.
- Take the first crust out and simply place evenly into the bottom of your pie pan.
- Add the coated apples to the piecrust, and spread them out into a nice heap.
- Place the butter pats evenly over the apples.
- Cover with the top with the other crust.

- Pinch down the edges of the top crust onto your pie pan. Then take a knife and make maybe 4 slits, lengthwise, at 12:00, 6:00, 3:00, and 9:00 in the crust.

Cooking the pie.
- If you just put the pie in the oven, the edges of the crust will burn. To prevent this, cover them with a couple of pieces of aluminum foil.
- Cook for 30 minutes at 375.
- Remove the foil and cook for another 15 minutes. Look to see when the crust begins to brown on top like in the cookbook photographs. At this point, it's ready.
- Be sure to let it cool a long time to let the apples set up. Otherwise, it'll goosh out all over the place when you try to cut it. This pie wants you to eat it with vanilla ice cream when it's still a little bit warm.

Note: A fantastic addition to this recipe is to mix in ½ cup walnut or ½ can of whole cranberries.

Banana Nut Bread

When Dottie and I first got together in graduate school, we had no money at all. We typically ended up scrounging around in the change jar for luxuries like food. Our apartment air conditioner blew hot air and water came out of our shower in a cross between a mist and a drizzle. We didn't even have chairs. But who needs these things when your bones still work and you can't stop looking at each other.

For Christmas, we couldn't afford to get our friends presents, so we baked. That's the "royal we." Dottie baked. I only sniffed from afar and pinched a taste whenever I could pull it off. The recipe below was the mainstay in our arsenal of Christmas goodies handed out to our friends. It was perfect because it basically uses cheap ingredients: nuts, flour, and rotten bananas.

You'll need:
<u>Dry Ingredients:</u>
> 3 ½ cups all-purpose flour
> 4 tsp baking powder
> ½ tsp baking soda
> 1 tsp salt
> 1 cup nuts

<u>Wet Ingredients:</u>
> ⅔ cup shortening
> 1 ⅓ cup sugar
> 4 eggs
> 2 cups ripe bananas

The dry bowl.
- Add in all dry ingredients into a bowl and mix well.

The wet bowl.
- Mash the shortening into the sugar until they're smooth.
- Add in the eggs. Beat them around until they're fluffy.
- Mash the bananas. Add them to the shortening, sugar, and eggs.

The twain shall meet.
- Take 1 cup of the dry ingredients and add them to the wet bowl. Stir until smooth. Keep doing this until you are out of dry ingredients.

Finishing up.
- Grease a bread pan with shortening, then sprinkle a bit of flour over the bottom.
- Bake at 350 for 45 minutes to 1 hour. A dry fork means it's done.

Raspberry Oatmeal Bars

This recipe comes to me courtesy of my dear friend Haley. The first time I read these ingredients, I remember thinking how decadent butter and brown sugar were together. I felt like I was getting away with something. Now, I feel like this is just the way things should be.

You'll need:
> 1 10 oz can raspberries from the freezer section
> 2 Tbsp cornstarch
> 2 Tbsp sugar
> ⅓ cup butter
> ⅔ cup brown sugar
> 1 tsp vanilla
> 1 cup oats
> 1 cup all purpose flour
> ½ tsp baking soda

Get the raspberries ready.
- First thaw the raspberries over medium heat. Add in cornstarch and sugar. Heat until it's thick and bubbly.

Get the crust together.
- Cream the butter and sugar together.
- Then add in the rest of the ingredients and blend them until it looks like coarse meal.
- Press 2 cups of this into an 8x8 pan.

Baking.
- Bake it for 12 minutes at 350.
- After it comes out, spread the raspberry mixture over the crust.
- Next, sprinkle it over with the remaining dry mixture.
- Bake for 15 minutes more.

Faux-Foods Quiz: Simpler is better

Memory is funny. I can't remember where I put my shoes, but I can tell you all the words to the Eagles Greatest Hits album I heard about a hundred years ago. I know the names of all my Elementary School teachers. It's as if my brain used to work, storing information into its long-term memory banks. But now my storer needs a lube job and a tune up.

When I read the ingredients of the product below, one of these ancient memories swims up from the bottom of some neural pool, breaking through the surface of my consciousness. "The fancier the plumbing, the easier it is to stop the drain." So says Mr. Scott – that wizened sage of the bowels of the Starship Enterprise. Incredibly complicated ingredient lists, like most faux-foods, include all kinds of strange things. Once you read the answer to this faux-food quiz, you'll wonder why in the world anyone would put propyl gallate in there, much less high-fructose corn syrup (the 2nd ingredient!). If Mr. Scott were a dietician, he would say, "The fancier the ingredient list, the easier it is to stop your drain."

Ingredients
Wheat flour, high-fructose corn syrup, dried onion, salt, partially hydrogenated soybean and/or cottonseed oils, hydrolyzed soy and corn protein, yeast, cooked chicken and chicken broth, soy flour, celery, maltodextrin, monosodium glutamate, whey, parsley flakes, spices, sugar, onion powder, caramel color, tumeric, di-sodium inosinate, di-sodium guanylate, sodium sulfite, BHA, BHT, propyl gallate, citric acid.

Hint
My mom makes this with cornbread (corn meal, buttermilk, an egg, and some baking soda). Now you tell me – when you see cornbread coming out of the oven, and its crunchy golden crust breaks open, and its soft middle drinks in the butter like a parched thirst downs a glass of water – what's better than that? Certainly not di-sodium inosinate.

APPENDIX

Resources for
Weight-Related Problems

American College of Nutrition
www.am-coll-nutr.org

American Diabetics Association
www.diabetes.org

American Dietetic Association
www.eatright.org

American Heart Association
www.americanheart.org

American Heart Association's Women's Web Site
women.americanheart.org

American Obesity Association
www.obesity.org

American Society for Clinical Nutrition
www.faseb.org/ascn

Center for Science in the Public Interest
www.cspinet.org/reports

Dietary Approaches to Stop Hypertension
dash.bwh.harvard.edu

Dietary Guidelines for Americans
www.nal.usdagov/fnic/dga/dguide95.html

Federal Obesity Clinical Guidelines
www.nih.gov/news/pr/jun98/nhlbi-17.htm

FDA Home Page (FDA)
www.fda.gov

Harvard School of Public Health
www.hsph.harvard.edu

Healthy School Meals Resource System
www.nal.usda.gov:8001

National Cancer Institute (NCI) Nutrition Implementation Group
www.dcp.nci.nih.gov/report/nutrition

National Institute for Diabetes and Digestive and Kidney Diseases
www.niddk.nih.gov

National Institutes of Health
text.nlm.nih.gov/nih

National Institutes of Health - Consensus Statements
odp.od.nih.gov/consensus

The New Food Label
vm.cfsan.fda.gov/~dms

NHLBI Obesity Guidelines
www.nhlbi.nih.gov/guidelines/obesity

The North American Association for the Study of Obesity
www.naaso.org

Obesity Law and Advocacy Center

www.obesitylaw.com

Obesity Surgery Journal
www.obesitysurgery.com
Oldways
www.oldwayspt.org

Physicians Committee for Responsible Medicine
www.pcrm.org

Statistics Related to Obesity
www.niddk.nih.gov/health/nutrit/pubs/statobes.htm

The Surgeon General of the United States
www.surgeongeneral.gov

U.S. Government health agencies
www.health.gov
www.healthfinder.gov

Weight Control Information Network
www.niddk.nih.gov/health

World Health Organization
www.who.int
www-nt.who.int/whosis/statistics

References on Mediterranean Diets

Books:

Allbaugh LG (1953): *Crete: A Case Study of an Underdeveloped Area.* Princeton, NJ: Princeton University Press.

Cloutier M, Adamson E (2001): *Mediterranean Diet.* Avon.

Emmerson M, Ewin J (Contributor) (1997): *The Healthy Feast: Cooking Light With Mediterranean Oils.* Inner Traditions Int Ltd.

Jenkins NH, Trichopoulou A (1994): *The Mediterranean Diet Cookbook : A Delicious Alternative for Lifelong Health.* Bantam Doubleday.

Jonas S, Gordon S (2000): *30 Secrets of the World's Healthiest Cuisines: Global Eating Tips and Recipes From China, France, Japan, the Mediterranean, Africa, and Scandinavia.* John Wiley & Sons

Keys A (1980): *Seven Countries: A Multivariate Analysis of Death and Coronary Heart Disease.* Cambridge, MA: Harvard University Press.

Perdue L (1992): *The French Paradox and Beyond: Live Longer with Wine and the Mediterranean Lifestyle.* Renaissance Publishing.

Ziff RA (1999): *Secrets of The French Diet.* Worldwide Publishing Inc.

Scientific Articles:

Boué C, Combe N, Billeaud C, Mignerot C, Entressangles B, Thery G, Geoffrion H, Brun JL, Dallay D, Leng JJ (2000): *Trans* Fatty acids in adipose tissue of French women in relation to their dietary sources. *Lipids 35* (5), pp. 561 – 566.

De Lorgeril M, Salen P (1999): Wine, ethanol, platelets, and Mediterranean diet. *Lancet 353*, p. 1067.

Ferro-Luzzi A, Sette S (1989): The Mediterranean Diet: An Attempt to Define its Present and Past Composition. *European Journal of Clinical Nutrition 43* (Supplement 2): pp. 13 – 29.

Kromhout D, Keys A, Aravanis C (1989): Food Consumption Patterns in the 1960s in Seven Countries. *American Journal of Clinical Nutrition 49*, pp. 889 – 894.

Willett WC (1994): Diet and Health: What Should We Eat? *Science 264*: pp. 532 – 7.

Willett WC (1997): Specific fatty acids and risks of breast and prostate cancer: dietary intake. *America Journal of Clinical Nutrition 66* (Suppl), pp. 1557s – 1563s.

World Health Organization. Food and Health Indicator in Europe. July 20, 1994 Nestle, M. (guest editor) Mediterranean diets: science and policy implications. *The American Journal of Clinical Nutrition*, 61:6(S). Supplement. Bethesda, MD: The American Society for Clinical Nutrition, Inc., June 1995.

The Role of Fat in Weight and Health

Books and Journals:

Barone A (2000): *Chic & Slim Encore: More About How French Women Dress Chic Stay Slim – and How You Can Too!* Nouvelles Editions

Bayan MJ, Carrea F (2000): *Eat Fat, Be Healthy: When A Low-Fat Diet Can Kill You.* Fireside.

Gittleman AL (1999): *Eat Fat, Lose Weight: How the Right Fats Can Make You Thin for Life.* Keats Publishing

Kass LR (1999): *The Hungry Soul: Eating and the Perfecting of Our Nature.* University of Chicago Press

Michael Fumento (1997): *The Fat of the Land: Our Health Crisis and How Overweight Americans Can Help Themselves.* Penguin Books

Payer L (1996): *Medicine & Culture.* Owl Books.

Pool R (2001): *Fat.* Oxford University Press.

Vigilante K, Flynn M (1999): *Low-Fat Lies, High-Fat Frauds: and The Healthiest Diet in the World.* Lifeline Press.

Weil A (2000): *Eating Well for Optimum Health.* Alfred A. Knopf.

The American Journal of Clinical Nutrition
    www.ajcn.org
    Supplements to this journal provide extremely informative reviews of the field or of particular aspects of the obesity epidemic.

International Journal of Obesity
    www.stockton-press.co.uk/ijo

Nutrition Science, Media, and Policy:

Basdevant A, Craplet C, and Guy-Grand B (1993): Snacking patterns in obese French women. *Appetite 21*, pp. 17 – 23.

Blair AJ (1991): When are calories most fattening? *Appetite 17*, p. 161.

Bufton MW (2000): Yesterday's science and policy: Diet and disease revisited. *Epidemiology 11* (4), pp. 474 – 476.

Hoebel BG (1997): Neuroscience and appetitive behavior research: 25 years. *Appetite 29*, pp. 119 – 133.

Marmot MG (1988): Diet and disease, and Durkheim and Dasgupta, and Deuteronomy. *Epidemiology 9*, pp. 676 – 680.

Mills M (1993): Expert policy advice to the British government on diet and heart disease. In Peters BG and Barker A (eds), *The Politics of Expert Advice: Creating, Using and Manipulating Scientific Knowledge for Public Policy*. Edinburgh: Edinburgh University Press.

Rozin P, Fischler C, Imada S, Sarubin A, and Wrzesniewski A (1999): Attitudes to food and the role of food in life in the U.S.A., Japan, Flemish Belgium, and France: Possible implications for the diet-health debate. *Appetite 33* (2), pp. 163 – 180.

Wellman NS, Scarbrough FE, Ziegler RG, and Lyle B (1999): Do we facilitate the scientific process and the development of dietary guidance when findings from single studies are publicized? *American Journal of Clinical Nutrition 70*, pp. 802 – 5.

Bariatric Surgery Articles:

Brolin RE, Bradley LJ, Wilson AC, Cody RP (2000): Lipid risk profile and weight stability after gastric restrictive operations for morbid obesity. *Journal of Gastrointestinal Surgery Sep-Oct 4*(5): pp. 464-9.

Deitel M (1998): Bariatric Surgery for Massive Obesity. *Acta Chir Austriaca 30*: pp. 149-153.

Goldberg S, Rivers P, Smith K, Homan W (2000): Vertical Banded Gastroplasty [colon] A Treatment for Morbid Obesity. *AORN Journal* 72(6) pp. 987-988, 991, 993, 995-1006, 1008-1010.

Bariatric Surgery Websites:

    American Society for Bariatric Surgery (ASBS)
        www.asbs.org
    The Center For Bariatric Surgery
        bariatricsurgeons.com
    Sociedad Española de Cirugía de la Obesidad (S.E.C.O)
        www.seco.org
    International College of Surgeons
        www.icsglobal.org
    International Federation for the Surgery of Obesity
        www.obesity-online.com/ifso

Liposuction Websites:

    www.plasticsurgery.org/faq/lipo.htm
    www.phudson.com/LIPOSUCTION/lipo.html
    www.liposite.com
    This site has liposuction discussion areas, searchable liposuction photo databases, and information about how to check on the credentials of your surgeon.

    www.drmelton.com/Chicago/Liposuction/lipo_home.html
    This site had a great deal of very valuable information on liposuction.

Diet and Cancer:

Doll R, Bingham SA (1981): The causes of cancer: Quantitative estimates of avoidable risks of cancer in the United States today. *Journal of the National Cancer Institute 66*, pp. 1191 – 1308.

Greenwald P, Milner JA, Clifford CK (2000): Creating a new paradigm in nutrition research within the National Cancer Institute. *Journal of Nutrition 130*, pp. 3103 – 3105.

Hart RW, Turturro A (1997): Dietary restriction and cancer. *Environmental Health Perspective 105*, pp. 989 – 992.

Kromhout D. (1987): Essential micronutrients in relation to carcinogenesis. *American Journal of Clinical Nutrition 45* (5 Suppl), pp. 1361-1367.

Willett WC (1999): Dietary fat and breast cancer. *Toxicological Science 52* (Suppl), pp. 127 – 146.

The Role of Vegetables:

Basdevant A, Craplet C, and Guy-Grand B (1993): Snacking patterns in obese French women. *Appetite 21*, pp. 17 – 23.

Blair AJ (1991): When are calories most fattening? *Appetite 17*, p. 161.

Kuo SM (1997): Dietary flavonoid and cancer prevention: Evidence and potential mechanism. *Critical Reviews in Oncology 8*, pp. 47 – 69.

Lee I-M (1999): Antioxidant vitamins in the prevention of cancer. *Proceedings of the Association of American Physicians 111*, pp. 10 – 15.

Ross (2000): Dietary flavonoids and the MLL gene: A pathway to infant leukemia? *Proceedings of the National Academy of Science USA, 97*, pp. 4411 – 4413.

Diet and Heart Disease:

National Research Council (U.S.) Committee on Diet and Health (1989): *Diet and Health: Implications for Reducing Chronic Disease Risk*. Washington, DC: National Academy Press.

De Lorgeril M, Salen P (1999): Wine ethanol, platelets, and Mediterranean diet. *Lancet 353*, p. 1067.

Hertog MGL, Kromhout D, Aravanis C, Blackburn H, Buzina R, Fidanza F, Giampaoli S, Jansen A, Menotti A, Nedeljkovic S (1995): Flavonoid intake and long-term risk of coronary heart disease and cancer in the Seven Countries Study. *Archives of Internal Medicine 155*, pp. 381 – 386.

Keys A (1952): The cholesterol problem. *Voeding 13*, pp. 539 – 555.

Keys A (ed) (1970): Coronary heart disease in seven countries. *Circulation 41* (Suppl 1).

Kromhout D (1999): Serum cholesterol in cross-cultural perspective: The Seven Countries study. *Acta Cardiologica 54* (3), pp. 151 – 158.

Marrugat J and Sentí S (2000): High cholesterol may not have same effect on cardiovascular risk in southern Europe as elsewhere. *Lancet 320*, p. 250.

Parodi PW (1997): The French paradox unmasked: The role of folate. *Medical Hypothesis 49*, pp. 313 – 318.

Renaud S, Berwick AD, Fehily AM, Sharp DS, and Elwood PC (1992): Alcohol and platelet aggregation: The Caerphilly prospective heart disease study. *American Journal of Clinical Nutrition 55*, pp. 1012 – 1017.

Rimm EB, Ellison RC (1995): Alcohol in the Mediterranean diet. *American Journal of Clinical Nutrition 61 (suppl)*, pp. 1378S – 1382S.

Steinberg D, Parthasarathy S, Carew TE, Khoo JC, Witzum JL (1989): Beyond cholesterol. Modifications of low-density lipoprotein that increase its atherogenicity. *New England Journal of Medicine 320*, pp. 915 – 924.

Tunstall-Pedoe H, Kuulasmaa K, Mähönen M, Tolonen H, Ruokokoski E, Amouyel P. (1999): Contribution of trends in survival and coronary-event rates to changes in coronary heart disease mortality: 10 year results from 37 WHO MONICA Project populations. *Lancet 353*, pp. 1547 – 1557.

Diet and the Metabolic Rate:

Almeras N, Lavallee N, Despres JP, Bouchard C, Tremblay A (1995): Exercise and energy intake: effect of substrate oxidation. *Physiological Behavior 57*, pp. 995 – 1000.

Dulloo AG, Jacquet J (1998): Adaptive reduction in basal metabolic rate in response to food deprivation in humans: A role for feedback signals from fat stores. *American Journal of Clinical Nutrition 86*, pp. 599 – 606.

Duffy PH, Feuers RJ, Nakamura KD, Leakey JA, Hart RW (1990): Effect of chronic caloric restriction on the synchronization of various physiological measures in old female Fischer-344 rats. *Chronobiology Int. 7*, pp. 113 – 124.

Duffy PH, Feuers RJ, Pipkin JL, Berg TF, Leakey JEA, Turturro A, Hart RW (1995): The effect of dietary restriction and aging on the physiological response of rodents to drugs. In (Hart RW et al., eds.) *Dietary Restriction: Implications for the Design and Interpretation of Toxicity and Carcinogenicity Studies.* pp. 127 – 141. ILSI Press: Washington, DC.

Goedecke JH, Christie C, Wilson G, Dennis SC, Noakes TD, Hopkins WG, Lambert EV (1999): Metabolic adaptations to a high-fat diet in endurance cyclists. *Metabolism 48* (12), pp. 1509 – 1517.

Hart RW, Dixit R, Seng J, Turturro A, Leakey JEA, Feuers R, Duffy P, Buffington C, Cowan G, Lewis S, Pipkin J, Li SY (1999): Adaptive role of caloric intake on the degenerative disease processes. *Toxicological Sciences 52* (Suppl), pp. 3 – 12.

Hill JO, Melanson EL (1999): Overview of the determinants of overweight and obesity: Current evidence and research issues. *Medicine and Science in Sports and Exercise 31* (11), pp. S515 – S521.

Hoppeler H, Billeter R, Horvath PJ, Leddy JJ, Pendergast DR (1999): Muscle structure with low- and high-fat diets in well-trained male runners. *International Journal of Sports Medicine 20* (8), pp. 522 – 526.

Horvath PJ, Eagen CK, Ryer-Calvin SD, Pendergast DR (2000): The effects of varying dietary fat on the nutrient intake in male and female runners. *Journal of the American College of Nutrition 19* (1), pp. 42 – 51.

Kris-Etherton PM, Pearson TA, Wan Y, Hargrove RL, Moriary K, Fishell V, and Etherton TD (1999): High-monounsaturated fatty acid diets lower both plasma cholestrol and triacylglycerol concentrations. *American Journal of Clinical Nutrition 70*, pp. 10009 – 10015.

Lavedrine F, Zmirou D, Ravel A, Balducci F, and Alary J (1999): Blood cholesterol and walnut consumption: A cross-sectional survey in France. *Preventative Medicine 28*, pp. 333 – 339.

Leakey JEA, Seng JE, Barnas CR, Baker VM, Hart RW (1998): A mechanistic basis for the beneficial effects of caloric restriction on longevity and disease: Consequences for the interpretation of rodent toxicity studies. *International Journal of Toxicology 17*, pp. 5 – 56.

Marmonier C, Chapelot D, and Sylvestre JL (1999): Metabolic and behavioral consequences of a snack consumed in a satiety state. *American Journal of Clinical Nutrition 70*, pp. 854-866.

Simi B, Sempore B, Mayet MH, Favier RJ (1991): Additive effects of training and high-fat diet on energy metabolism during exercise. *Journal of Applied Physiology 71*, pp. 197 – 203.

Wadden TA, Itallie TB, Blackburn GL (1990): Responsible and irresponsible use of very-low-calorie diets in the treatment of obesity. *Journal of the American Medical Association 263*, pp. 83 – 85.

Diet and Faux-Foods

Reviews:

American Academy of Pediatrics (1985): Committee on Drugs, "Inactive" ingredients in pharmaceutical products. *Pediatrics 76*, pp. 635 – 643.

Smith JM, Dodd TRP (1982): Adverse reactions to pharmaceutical excipients. *Adverse Drug React Acute Pois Rev 1*, pp. 93 – 142.

Weiner M, Bernstein IL (1989): *Adverse Reactions to Drug Formulation Agents: A Handbook of Excipients.* New York: Marcel Dekker, Inc.

Websites:

www.hsph.harvard.edu/Academics/nutr/olestra
www.cspinet.org/reports/food.htm
www.cspinet.org/additives

Dyes:

Caucino JA, Armenaka M, Rosenstreich DL (1994): Anaphylaxis associated with a change in premarin dye formulation. *Annals of Allergy 72*, pp. 33 – 35.

Hunt LW, Dunn WF (1991): Anaphylaxis following a Kenalog (triamcinolone acetonide) injection: hypersensitivity to carboxymethyl-cellulose. *Journal of Allergy and Clinical Immunology 87*, p. 277.

Lockey SD (1971): Reaction to hidden agents in foods, beverages, and drugs. *Annals of Allergy 29*, pp. 461 – 466.

Malanin G, Kalimo K (1989): The results of skin testing with food additives and the effect of an elimination diet in chronic and recurrent urticaria and recurrent angioedema. *Clinics of Experimental Allergy 19*, pp. 539 – 543.

Aspartame:

Blaylock RL (1996): *Excitotoxins: The Taste That Kills.* Health Press.

Ikonomidou C, Mosinger JL, Shahid Salles K, Labruyere J, Olney JW (1989): Sensitivity of the developing rat brain to hypobaric/ischemic damage parallels sensitivity to N-Methyl-Aspartate neurotoxicity. *Journal of Neuroscience 9*, pp. 2809 – 2818.

Kretchmer N, Hollenbeck CB (eds.) (1991): *Sugars and Sweeteners.* Boca Raton: CRC Press, pp. 151-167, 232-237.

McDonald JW, Silverstein FS, Johnston MV (1988): Neurotoxicity of NMDA is markedly enhanced in developing rat central nervous system. *Brain Research 459*, pp. 200 – 203.

Olney JW (1969): Brain lesions, obesity and other disturbances in mice treated with monosodium glutamate. *Science 164*, pp. 719 – 721.

Olney JW (1984): Excitotoxic food additives – relevance of animal studies to human safety. *Neurobehavioral Toxicology and Teratology 6*, pp. 455 – 462.

Olney JW (1994): Excitotoxins in foods. *Neurotoxicology 15* (3), pp. 535 – 544.

Reynolds WA, Lemkey-Johnston N, Filer LJ, Pitkin RM (1971): Monosodium glutamate: absence of hypothalamic lesions after ingestion by newborn primates. *Science 172*, 1342 – 1344.

Smith JM (1991): Adverse reactions to food and drug additives. *European Journal of Clinical Nutrition 45* [Suppl 1], pp. 17 – 21.

Stegink LD, Reynolds WA, Filer LJ, Pitkin R, Boaz DP, Brummer MC (1975): Monosodium glutamate metabolism in the neonatal monkey. *American Journal of Physiology 229*, pp. 246 – 250.

Wang GJ, Labruyere J, Price MT, Olney JW (1990): Extreme sensitivity of infant animals to glutamate toxicity: Role of NMDA receptors. *Neuroscience Abstracts 16*, p. 198.

See Also:
www.invisibledisabilities.com/nutrabomb.htm
www.healthproducts.cc/news-aspartame.htm
tc.engr.wisc.edu/tcweb/uer/uer98/wahlen.html
www.sunsentpress.com/aspartamekills.com
www.swankin-turner.com/aspartame/hist.html

High-Fructose Corn Syrup:

Holbrook JT, Smith JC, Reiser S (1989): Dietary fructose or starch: effects on copper, zinc, iron, manganese, calcium, and magnesium balances in humans. *American Journal of Clinical Nutrition 49*, pp. 1290 – 1294.

Ivaturi R, Kies C (1992): Mineral balances in humans as affected by fructose, high-fructose corn syrup and sucrose. *Plant Foods for Human Nutrition 42*, pp. 143 – 151.

Kumar A, Aitas AT, Hunter AG, Beaman DC (1996): Sweeteners, dyes, and other excipients in vitamin and mineral preparations. *Clinical Pediatrics Sept*, pp. 443 – 450.

Lingelback LB, McDonald RB (2000): Description of the long-term lipogenic effects of dietary carbohydrates in male Fischer 344 rats. *Journal of Nutrition 130*, pp. 3077 – 3084.

Milne DB, Nielsen FH (2000): The interaction between dietary fructose and magnesium adversely affects macromineral homeostasis in men. *Journal of the American College of Nutrition 19* (1), pp. 31 – 37.

Park KY, Yetley EA (1993): Intakes and food sources of fructose in the United States. *American Journal of Clinical Nutrition 58* (Suppl), pp. 737S – 747S.

Reiser S, Powell AS, Scholfield DJ, Panda P, Ellwood KC, Canary JJ (1989): Blood lipids, lipoproteins, apoproteins, and uric acid in men fed diets containing fructose or high-amylose cornstarch. *American Journal of Clinical Nutrition 49*, pp. 832 – 839.

Swanson JE, Laine DC, Thomas W, Bantle JP (1992): Metabolic effects of dietary fructose in healthy subjects. *American Journal of Clinical Nutrition 55*, pp. 851 – 856.

Answers to Faux-Food Quizzes

1. **What are faux-foods?** (p. 9)
   CoffeeMate non-dairy creamer
2. **Kids**
   Hellmann's 97% Fat Free Mayonnaise Dressing (p. 29)
3. **Stealth food products** (p. 45)
   Kool-Aid Lemonade
4. **Paints, plastics, and glues. Oh my!** (p. 63)
   General Foods International Coffees: French Vanilla Café
5. **Picture this** (p. 77)
   Hershey's Lite Syrup
6. **Good try-ers** (p. 93)
   a. Jalenpeño cheese spread
   b. Fat Free Cheese Food
   c. Better 'n Eggs "Egg product"
7. **Naugahyde** (115)
   Domino's Pizza Garlic Sauce
8. **Great kid afternoons** (p. 139)
   Cheetoes
9. **It's on your pie** (p. 161)
   Cool Whip
10. **A test for spies** (p. 179)
    Reduced Fat Peanut Butter (Compare this with the ingredients in Smuckers Peanut Butter: Peanuts)
11. **Fool me once, shame on you** (p. 195)
    Little Debbie Swiss Rolls
12. **A little sugar, sweetie?** (p. 207)
    a. Hot dog relish
    b. Heinz Catsup
    c. Hotdog Buns
    d. Coca-Cola
13. **Simpler is better** (p. 245)
    Stove Top Stuffing

Index

D

Quick Order Form on Reverse

Perusal Press

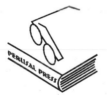

PO Box 408
North Versailles, PA 15137

The Fat Fallacy: Quick Order Form

For general information on buying *The Fat Fallacy* or attending a workshop in your area, **see the FatFallacy.com website!**
Price: $24.95 US + $3.00 Shipping & Handling

Please send me a copy of *The Fat Fallacy: Applying the French Diet to the American Lifestyle*. I understand that I may return this book for a full refund – for any reason, no questions asked.

Email orders: willclower@fatfallacy.com
For Postal orders:
Please fill out this form and send to:
      Perusal Press
      PO Box 408
      North Versailles, PA 15137

Name: _____

Email Address: _____

Postal Address: _____

City: _____ State: _____ Zip: _____

Telephone: _____

Payment: **Check**

              Credit: Visa, MasterCard, AMEX, Discover

Card Number: _____

Name on Card: _____

Exp. Date:____/____

Signature: _____

<u>Quick Order Form on Reverse</u>

Perusal Press

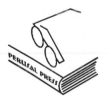

PO Box 408
North Versailles, PA 15137

The Fat Fallacy: <u>Quick Order Form</u>

For general information on buying *The Fat Fallacy* or attending a workshop in your area, **see the FatFallacy.com website!**
Price: $24.95 US + $3.00 Shipping & Handling

Please send me a copy of *The Fat Fallacy: Applying the French Diet to the American Lifestyle*. I understand that I may return this book for a full refund – for any reason, no questions asked.

Email orders: willclower@fatfallacy.com
For Postal orders:
Please fill out this form and send to:
      Perusal Press
      PO Box 408
      North Versailles, PA 15137

Name: _____
Email Address: _____
Postal Address: _____
City: _____ State: _____ Zip: _____
Telephone: _____

Payment: <u>Check</u>

           <u>Credit:</u> Visa, MasterCard, AMEX, Discover
Card Number: _____
Name on Card: _____
Exp. Date:____/____
Signature: _____

Quick Order Form on Reverse

Perusal Press

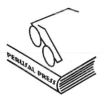

PO Box 408
North Versailles, PA 15137

The Fat Fallacy: <u>Quick Order Form</u>

For general information on buying *The Fat Fallacy* or attending a workshop in your area, **see the FatFallacy.com website!**
Price: $24.95 US + $3.00 Shipping & Handling

Please send me a copy of *The Fat Fallacy: Applying the French Diet to the American Lifestyle*. I understand that I may return this book for a full refund – for any reason, no questions asked.

Email orders: willclower@fatfallacy.com
For Postal orders:
Please fill out this form and send to:
      Perusal Press
      PO Box 408
      North Versailles, PA 15137

Name: _____

Email Address: _____

Postal Address: _____

City: _____ State: _____ Zip: _____

Telephone: _____

Payment: <u>Check</u>

           <u>Credit:</u> Visa, MasterCard, AMEX, Discover

Card Number: _____

Name on Card: _____

Exp. Date:____/____

Signature: _____